A Stroke of Poetry

To my father and my inspiration

Gerald McGowan
(1934 – 2007)

Acknowledgements

Many thanks to all my family and friends, both in Australia and the UK, who have supported me tremendously through my stroke recovery.

Karen Bayly, Heather Tutweiler and Ida Dempsey who became my good friends through the *FAST parenting after a stroke* Facebook page, and provided invaluable advice in understanding the emotions after suffering stroke. Thank you for urging me to get my poems in print.

Carol and Bob Bridgestock, crime writers and friends who posted some of my early poems on their blog and provided great advice in getting started with my book.
blog.rcbridgestock.com/?p=2010

I am grateful to artists Sharon Morgan and Georgina Westley for their contribution in the form of artwork for you to colour and to encourage creativity.

Diana Kerr and many others from the National Stroke Foundation who never cease to care about my stroke journey and always have the time to talk, and most importantly listen and provide advice where needed.

To Alex Mitchell of Author Support Services, my fabulous editor, without whose expertise and guidance this book would not have been possible.

A Stroke of Poetry

Poems of healing and hope after stroke

Shelagh Brennand

A Stroke of Poetry
Author – Shelagh Brennand

© Shelagh Brennand 2015

Astrokeofpoetry@gmail.com
www.astrokeofpoetry.com

This publication is sold with the understanding that the author is not offering specific personal advice to the reader. This publication is not intended as a substitute for the professional or medical advice of a suitable, qualified practitioner.

The author disclaims any responsibility for liability, loss or risk, personal or otherwise, that happens as a consequence of the use and application of any of the contents of this publication.

This publication may not be reproduced in whole or part, stored, posted on the internet, or transmitted in any form or by any means, electronic, mechanical, photocopying, recording, or other, without permission from the author of this publication. All rights reserved.

Colouring artwork:
  Sharon Morgan www.manifestingmandalas.com
  Georgina Westley www.georginawestley.co.uk

Back cover photo:
  Lou O'Brien www.imagesbylouobrien.com

Editing and consultation:
  Alex Mitchell www.AuthorSupportServices.com

Design: Sylvie Blair www.bookpod.com

National Library of Australia Cataloguing-in-Publication entry
Creator: Brennand, Shelagh, author.
Title: A stroke of poetry: poems of healing and hope after stroke / Shelagh Brennand
ISBN: 9780994162922 (paperback)   9780994162953 (e-book)
Subjects: Healing – Poetry
              Hope – Poetry
              Cerebrovascular disease – Poetry
Dewey Number: A821.4

Foreword

Stroke is a devastating event for those who survive it, and the effects extend far beyond the immediately visible paralysis and communication problems. Disabling fatigue, difficulty with concentrating and thinking, and emotional problems are unseen from the outside, but extremely common and often the most disabling and distressing sequelae for the stroke survivor. Medicine is only beginning to understand just how important this is, and we have a long way to go in developing effective interventions.

The good news is that recovery, though usually a long process, is possible. We do know that physical, social, and mental activity is extremely important in the recovery phase, and Shelagh's journey is an excellent example of this. She has embraced the experience of her stroke in a positive way and used the creative outlet of poetry and the compilation of this book as part of her recovery. I commend this book, especially for anyone who is struggling with unseen effects following a health challenge. Take Shelagh's words and example as an inspiration and stimulus to accept and rise above your personal challenges.

Dr Rohan Grimley, Stroke Physician

Contents

> Stroke kills more men than prostate cancer.

Introduction 2

Not me – I'm only 49! 6

My history 11

The Stroke Foundation network 13

My poems 17

I understand 21

Mornings 26

My thoughts, poems and artwork 29

Who stole my brain? 33

Homework time 37

A visit to the principal 38

Post stroke depression 44

My thoughts, poems and artwork 47

Muffin maker extraordinaire 52

Down day 57

I want to climb a mountain 63

Feeling low 64

> 1 in 6 people will have a stroke.

Financial advisor phobia 73

I wish I had wings 74

Our Lilly 81

Six months on 82

It's only oranges 84

Non-working mum 86

My thoughts, poems and artwork 89

The party animal no more 93

The luckiest wife in the world 94

School holidays 99

The inflatables 101

End of challenge thankyou 103

Climbing mountains now 108

I did it! 112

Ding-a-lingin' 114

Happy, two years on 116

What now? 122

> 20 percent of people who experience a stroke are under the age of 55.

> Post-stroke fatigue affects between 40 and 70 percent of stroke survivors.

> The good news is that most strokes are preventable.

> Stroke is one of Australia's biggest killers and a leading cause of disability.

Introduction

I was a busy wife and mum, working as an independent Private Investigator. This was my retirement job, having previously served 25 years as a UK Police Officer.

On 15 April 2013, I suffered a stroke and my whole life changed. I am now what many people refer to as a 'stroke survivor'. However I am much more than my condition. My name is Shelagh and I live in Queensland, Australia with my lovely husband David and son Patrick.

I was lucky enough to be left with no physical disability after the initial problems of loss of speech, and loss of feeling in my right side, dissipated. I still suffer from daily fatigue, but know I got off lightly.

Post stroke, I discovered my brain had changed. It seemed to function well in rhyme and most of my thoughts could not be processed unless the end of each sentence rhymed. I began to write down my thoughts and emotions in the form of poetry and soon learnt these feelings were not just experienced by me, but are shared by many stroke survivors. It was refreshing and comforting to know that I was never alone during my recovery.

These poems are about my day to day experiences; the thoughts, struggles and triumphs of my recovery as a stroke survivor. They are set out chronologically, following my journey through times of despair and depression, back to a normal life. The stroke recovery was a roller coaster of mixed emotions but being able to document in poetry even the darkest moments kept me motivated and gave me a will to carry on.

By writing, I could express myself and release the negative and frustrating emotions, and by looking back over the poems I soon realised that as these darker moments passed, each day became brighter. I hope that upon reading them, you can read the struggle but also accept the triumphs which now far outweigh the negativity.

You may feel some of the poems are confronting, and they may well be, as I wrote them to help release negative emotions such as sadness, frustration, post stroke depression and the utter feeling of despair. Other poems detail the funniest moments of forgetfulness and mishap, but all the poems are entirely true.

When I review them now I can see how important it was to maintain a positive mindset and a healthy, active life. With those two ground rules, I feel I have shown myself that anything is possible.

Along my own journey, many have asked me how to stay motivated during the frustration and depression that is so common post-stroke. This has always been a difficult question to answer, but I do believe that creativity has been a key for me. Poetry has been my own creative outlet, but we are all different. Some of us like to write, some to draw and some to paint. The use of colour therapy is regarded by many as a powerful tool to aid healing.

I've added some pages within the book for you to colour in, to express yourself in your own way. I hope this also adds some light to the 'darker' poems. There are also a few pages where you could write your own poems, or doodles, or drawing. Why not have a go exploring your own creativity.

Some of these poems were posted on the *FAST parenting after a stroke* Facebook site, and the first poem, of events on the day of the stroke, was published in the Spring 2013 issue of *Stroke Connection*, a newsletter sent to thousands of stroke survivors and their families around Australia.

Please enjoy my poems as much as I have enjoyed writing them. If you are reading as a stroke survivor, or on behalf of a loved one, I trust they give you some hope and positivity, helping you through the day with the knowledge you are not alone.

www.astrokeofpoetry.com

Stroke kills more women than breast cancer.

A bird sitting on a tree is never afraid of the branch breaking, because her trust is not on the branch but on its own wings. Always believe in yourself.

Author unknown

Not me – I'm only 49!

'Twas a sunny day in Queensland, the day that changed my life.
How was I to know a little gardening would cause us all such strife?
The day before I'd been with friends, and really feeling great.
49 and fit as can be, and I'd even lost some weight.

The last day of the holidays, I cherished with my son.
We weeded, seeded, trimmed and chopped, until it all was done.
"Please can I now go inside?" he asked with a frown.
So that left me in the garden, lawn mowing on my own.

The day was hot, I'd done a lot, and I should have taken a break.
So I went inside to have a rest, perhaps a meal to make.
I suddenly came over all dizzy, hot and a little squiffy.
My head into the toilet, I thought would sort it in a jiffy.

That's the last thing I remember, before I clearly fell.
When I awoke I saw my son and didn't feel too well.
His name that I first shouted, I could say no more.
I could not move a muscle, from that cold, hard bathroom floor.

My mouth it moved, but no words came, I thought I had gone dumb.
My right leg couldn't move at all, my right side had gone numb.
Oh his little face, I see it still every day.
Such calm, then panic looking at me, slumped in disarray.

A friend, thank goodness, came around and knew just what to do.
The next thing I remember was the marvellous ambulance crew.
"A stroke," they muttered to themselves, I thought it could not be
In three months' time I would be only half a century.

"I'm far too young, you've got it wrong," I thought and tried to say.
I couldn't be a stroke victim, on that lovely sunny day.
The words, the tubes, the tests and things they had to do.
Scared, confused and helpless, but that crew, they got me through.

The flashing lights at every stop, the sirens and the rush.
Could this be really happening to me, a 49 year old lush?
The hospital, now that was fun, the chaos and the mayhem.
Those doctors they worked tirelessly, I could never be one of them.

The days that followed had good news, the stroke team did their bit.
A clot had caused this sorry mess and soon I would be fit.
My voice came back quite easily, and soon my walking too.
I knew I was a lucky girl, despite the hullabaloo.

So now this brings me three months on and wow have I improved,
Though fatigue still racks my head and my body too.
"Don't rush back to your old life," advice it came in droves.
Since I've been well I seem to have a brain so full of odes.

These poems are the strangest thing; they swirl around in my head.
Quite often, I just cannot sleep and must get out of bed.
My social worker, what a lady, Judy was so great.
She said the brain does wondrous things; don't fight them, celebrate.

I'm 50 now, I got there quick, with friends to roust me on.
A husband, sister close at hand and of course my loving son.
The recovery months are still to come, so rest is still a key.
Who knows what lies ahead for us, life is a mystery.

So please take note of my young age, for this tale it is so true.
Just be aware of your own limits, or it can happen to you.

*You can't start a
new chapter
of your life
if you keep re-reading
the last one.*

Michael McMillan

My history

My name is Shelagh, that you know, I'm sure there's more to tell.
I had my stroke two years ago but most days I feel quite well.
I live in sunny Queensland, with my 'nearly' 14 year old son.
My husband had a FIFO job during my stroke, which wasn't fun.

We immigrated seven years ago, a business visa was our thing.
My husband set things up from scratch, his business data cabling.
After months of 'ladies that lunch' it was time to get off my bum.
So I got my PI's licence, and that really has been fun.

I was a UK cop for 25 years, so this was something I could do.
Investigations, loved them all 'til my stroke, and now my brain is goo!
No physical ailments do I have, except this terrible fatigue.
But brain ache, migraines, although now much less, are definitely in my league.

Most days I'm fine, I function well, and feel quite positive.
But when those bad days came, I felt I could not live.
The mental thing, it got me down, when those days, they had no meaning.
Then a few days hence, they'd gone again, so weird, but so relieving.

My brain won't work the same just yet, but maybe it will in time.
To keep myself so occupied, I tend to write everything in rhyme.
I've poems stored up, in my silly brain, and some I've just let go.
About my life since I had my stroke, so enjoy them as you go.

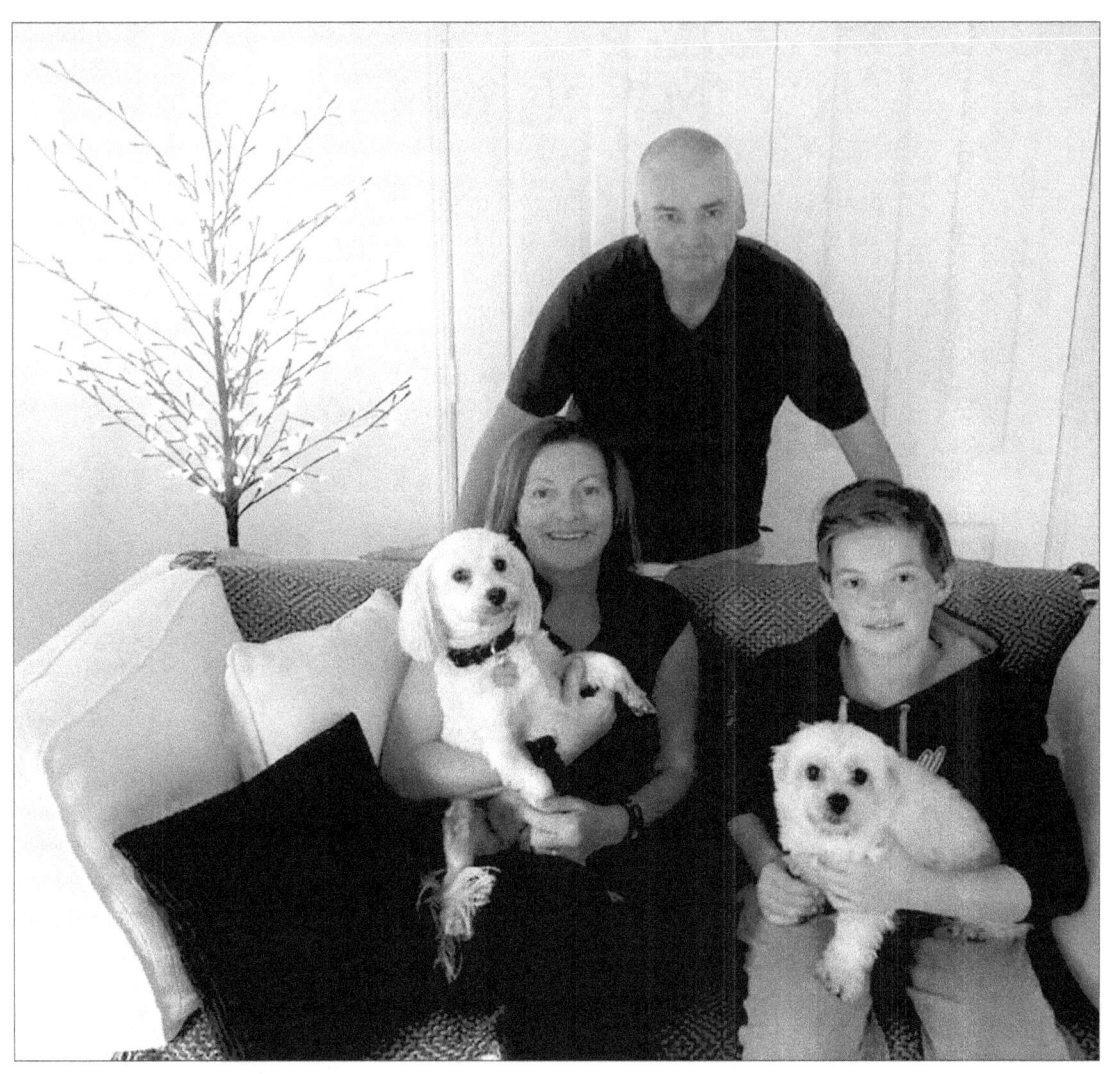

The Stroke Foundation network

Now I'm in hospital, pray who do I tell?
How can I communicate that I'm not very well?
I know my friends will be concerned; I know that they all care.
But I also know the Shelagh that was, and she's no longer there.

It's hard to think, it's hard to know, and how to tell my news.
When in reality I'm not so happy; I have the post stroke blues.
So who is close, who do I tell? Perhaps they should know first.
Facebook? No, I don't think so yet, too early for such an outburst.

Family, close friends and those so near, the tale I had to tell.
They all were shocked, and sad and mad because I'd seemed so well.
You're fit, and not yet 50, they all said with horror as they spoke.
But as I've learned recently, it can happen to any folk.

I've had support from so far and wide and Facebook now it's on.
The Stroke Foundation spoke with me, giving me faith to carry on.
My stroke friends from around the world, they make me cry and laugh.
Our dizzy tales of things we do, make me realise I'm not alone, or daft.

I feel so proud of what I've achieved, only a few months on.
And know that I have steps to take, to help me carry on.
So thank you everyone, for your support and keeping me so strong.
At last, I feel quite comfortable and know where I belong.

My old life's gone, that is OK, I now do understand.
I think my new life will be fun and no doubt in some ways grand.
So 'til next time, love to all, and hope your day is good
You're all so strong, you know you are, so give yourselves a hug

*Sometimes we need
someone to be there.
Not to fix anything,
or to do anything in particular,
but just to let us feel that we are
cared for and supported.*

Author unknown

My poems

I love to write my poems, I write them day and night.
I know the rhyming is terrible, and they never sound quite right.

I really can't stop writing them; I do it all day long.
I know there are other things to do, but is this pastime wrong?

I've no idea why I write them, my brain just tells me so.
And why not, my gorgeous social worker said, give anything a go.

I need to keep my brain intact, as these days it's rather slow.
So these poems help me work my brain and keep me on the go.

I cannot play the piano and a song I cannot sing.
So I've decided that maybe these poems are my thing.

They are not hurting anyone, though my husband thinks I'm mad.
I think that if you ask him, he will say my poems are quite bad.

Awful headaches seem to come and go each day.
But when I write my poems, it washes them away.

My exploits since the stroke I've had, some sad and some just weird.
I write them down in Pam Ayres style and then I can be heard.

Some things I do, they're so bizarre, I really can't explain.
I'm sure that we all know by now, we have a complex brain.

I really hope you like them but if you don't, that's fine by me.
But if they helped me get through this, that's good, you will agree.

So, off I go to write some more, the dishes they can wait.
And enjoy the day and what's in store, and life to celebrate.

ENJOY
the little things in life.
For some day you will
look back and realise
they were the BIG things.

Robert Brault

I understand

Please don't talk to me in baby talk. It really isn't good.
Even though my words don't come out right, I can hear; I understood.

Don't finish all my sentences. When you talk to me this way,
it's clear you wish I'd hurry up so we can get on with the day.

Even though my words are jumbled and I slur to get them out,
inside I know what I want to say so give me time and please don't shout.

It's important for me to process what I think I want to tell.
Even though when the words are spoken, they may not come out too well.

Buckets of patience I know you'll need to help me through this time.
But please, oh please be mindful, they are not your words but mine.

I know my brain will heal but you have to give me space.
Having a conversation does not need to be a race.

Sometimes I may not want to join in what anyone has to say.
But that's okay, I do not mind, as my brain needs a rest today.

*Every day
may not be good…
BUT
there is something good
in every day.*

Alice Morse Earle

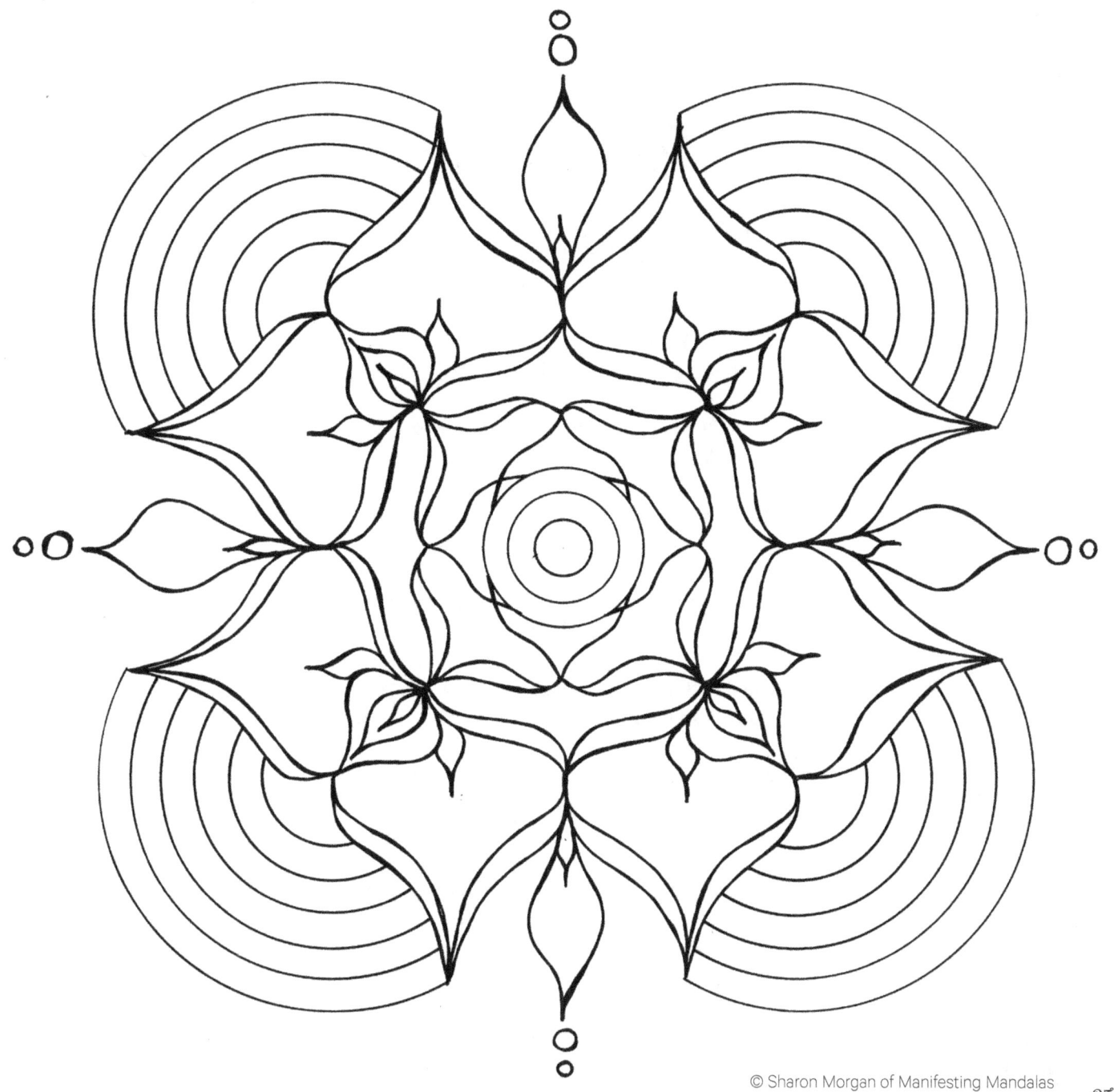

Mornings

Today I woke up weary,
and perhaps a little teary.

Do I have to get out of bed?
The dog and my son, they need to be fed.

I have to budge, I have to move.
C'mon Shelagh, get with the groove.

The shower goes on, mine, not that of my son.
I shout to Patrick to get a move on.

Is it pancakes for brekkie, or a cereal fix?
It's a breakfast shake, that sugary mix.

You'd better get dressed and your bags to pack.
Did you brush your teeth, why are they looking black?

A frantic search for our lovely pup,
while my peppermint tea goes cold in my cup.

Lock the house, get in the car.
Thank goodness we don't have to go very far.

We're in the car, and off we go.
Is the house locked? Where did Lilly go?

Before my stroke was I ever this bad.
A frantic mum and her disorganised lad.

Maybe I did it all for him before.
But as I keep reminding him, he's no longer four!

So I drop him off, on time today.
And back home I go, to disarray.

The beds now made, the washing done.
Perhaps today I will have some fun?

Maybe I'll sit and ponder a while.
And wait until pick up to see his smile.

Then it's post school business, rushing around.
Tomorrow, will my organised brain be found?

My thoughts, poems and artwork

*It does not matter
how slowly you go,
as long as
you do not stop.*

Confucius

Who stole my brain?

Some days I sit and wonder whose brain I've got.
I used to be intelligent - and now I'm clearly not!
On the day I had my stroke, my brain it did get taken.
And replaced with a mixed up one, that makes me feel forsaken.

My new brain, it won't settle well, it doesn't like my head.
It won't let me do the things I did, and makes me stay in bed.
My new brain is all over the place, and often makes me late.
When will I get used to my new brain and be able to think things straight?

Maybe I'll start to like my new brain, and hopefully one day soon.
Even though I'm asleep at half past four on sunny afternoons.
My new brain taps into different parts of me I'd never found
and maybe thinks of things to do that one day make me proud.

You know I do these silly rhymes, I don't think that is amazing.
So I really hope I'll do something else or these will drive me crazy.
Should I accept my new brain, or should I try to fight it?
Should I try to get my old one back and see if I still like it?

My old brain was so full of ideas, and always on the go.
So perhaps my new brain isn't all bad, and it's trying to tell me so.
Then stop looking for my old brain, someone else can have it.
And I will stick with my new brain for now, and hope one day it will fit.

To those with new brains, I know they're hard to fit,
but to the brain thief out there, you're most welcome to it.

At the end of the day tell yourself gently, "I love you. You did the best you could today, and even if you didn't accomplish all you had planned, I love you anyway".

Francois

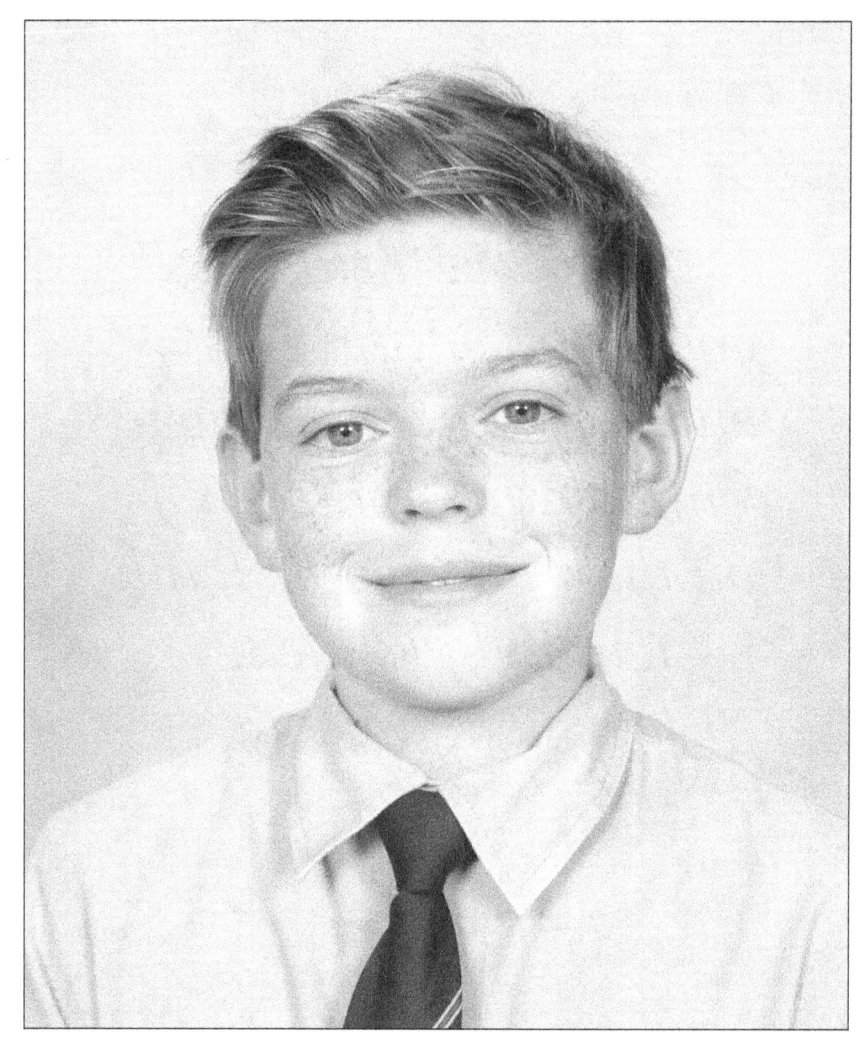

Homework time

Oh no, it's that awful time again, when Patrick's homework comes a calling.
I have this fear and awful dread, as my concentration is appalling.

I try to check he knows his stuff, but I really have no clue.
This stroke left me without an idea of really what to do.

I sit with him, and offer help, and scary as it may seem,
he looks at me with his loving eyes and I think I'm in a dream.

I used to help, and offer advice, and know just how it went.
But now at the end of a tiring day, my energy is spent.

"You'll work it out," I have to say, as the answer I don't know.
I feel helpless, useless, a terrible mum, but try not to let my feelings show.

But you know what happens, after all that, he completes it on his own.
My inadequacies as usual, I seem to not have shown.

I hate this feeling of not being useful, or being able to help him out.
But every day I do my best, and for that there is no doubt.

If we can't be like we were before, then we shouldn't give a damn.
What's important is that we do our best and just do what we can.

A visit to the principal

Today it is the visit I had put off since last May.
I have to go alone today as David works away.
Patrick got the scholarship for next year in Grade Eight.
He's such a clever chap, my son, only five more months to wait.

The results of the exam are with the principal Dr D.
But they need to be explained today, and now there's only me.
Well, my brain capacity, it can't take on complex things.
So iPad charged and off I go, we shall see what this day brings.

I sit in her big office, awaiting now my fate.
It's now just gone six minutes to three, and here I fret and wait.
I feel like a nervous schoolgirl, waiting for the cane.
I wish I wasn't by myself with my poor old damaged brain.

She finally enters with a smile and a lovely, warm handshake too.
She is a lovely lady, I wish my brain was not like goo!
She asks me how I'm doing and she listens with intent.
The past few months I then recount and how they have been spent.

We chat, we laugh then look at Patrick's complex data sheet.
I look at it but don't know what it means. Do I admit defeat?
The info is too much for me; it gives me such a fright.
I need my helpful iPad to ensure I've got it right.

So I pull it from my big bag, flying out with tissues and gum.
I really feel a silly, stupid, incompetent mum.
I open up the iPad, I try to switch it on.
But then I suddenly realise, the battery is all gone.

I thought back to when I'd charged it, and recall the plug I'd used.
Clearly, I had done this wrong, and I wasn't now amused.
Please can I have some paper, and notes I'd have to write.
I'm slowly sinking into my chair as this may take all night.

But actually, I surprised myself, few notes I had to make.
I listened now intently so to avoid any mistakes.
Our son had done remarkably in the subjects that he'd taken.
His results they were outstanding; an A student in the making.

After half an hour, all the info now I'd gotten.
So I rushed straight home to type it out, for fear of it being forgotten.
The moral of this story, I'm sure you know it well.
Have confidence in what you do....and charge your iPad well!

*A certain darkness
is needed
to see the stars.*

Osho

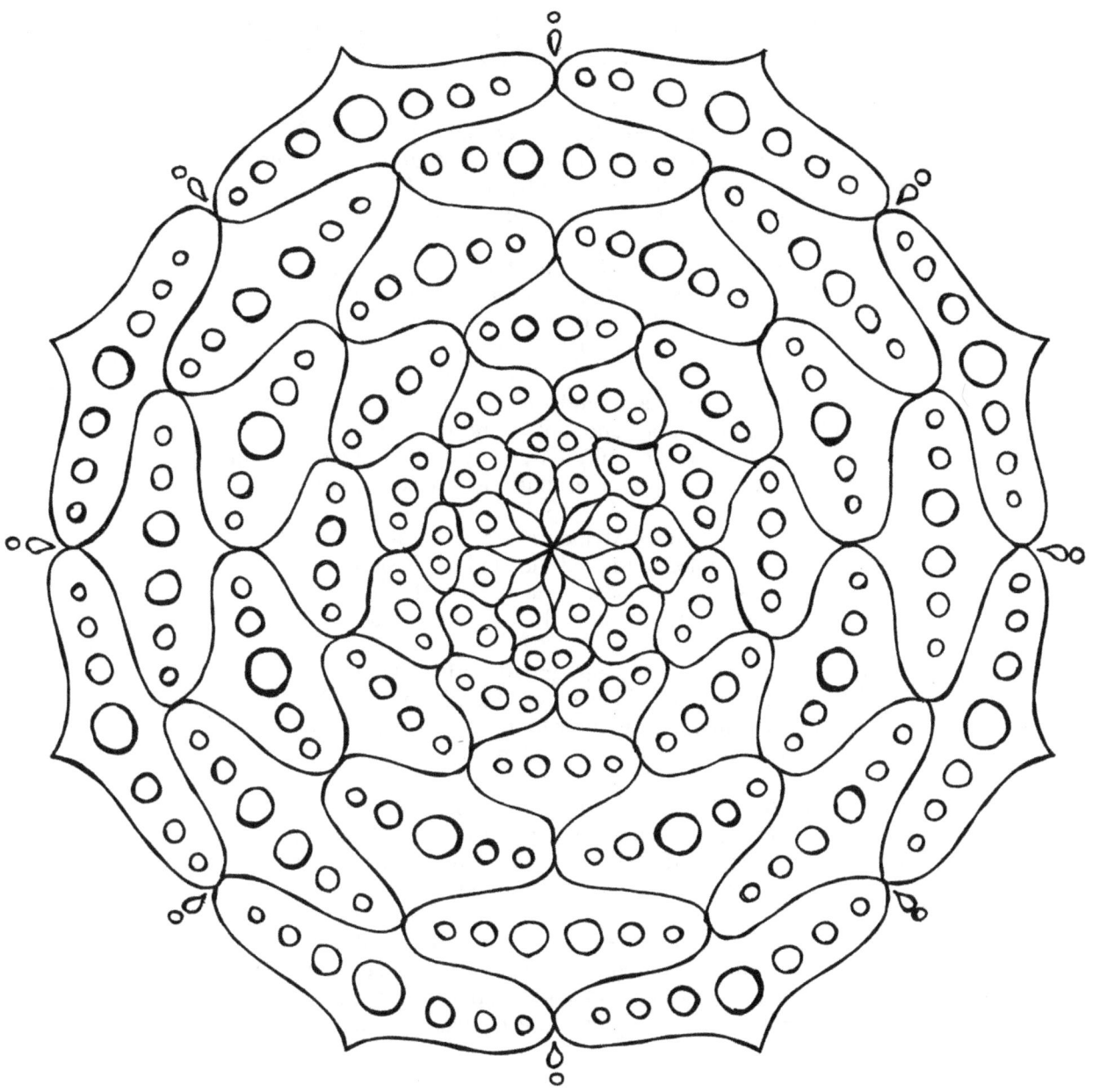

© Sharon Morgan of Manifesting Mandalas
Used with permission.

Post stroke depression

'Post stroke depression', my consultant warned me.
Please will you watch out for it, the stats are two in three.
'Post stroke depression', I laughed back in his face.
I'm going to tackle this stroke with vigour and with grace.

Initially I was fed up, but I'll ask you, who wouldn't be?
My life had changed so drastically, my old life no longer to be.
Two months after, I flew to England, my son with me all the way.
My nephew he got married, I could not miss his wedding day.

We caught up with friends and lots of family in those two weeks.
I listened to my body and took my needed rest in between.
Three months on was my birthday, many celebrations to be done.
A party, lots of friends around and I had a heap of fun.

My husband took me to Melbourne and a smashing time we had.
We ate, we drank and relaxed a lot and there was nothing bad.
I still rested in amongst the laughter of this happy time.
I really felt I was getting well; no depression on my mind.

Then four months on, my husband, he returned to his work away.
I don't know what the trigger was but I began to feel dismay.
Perhaps now all the festivities had been and gone in a short time.
I suddenly felt so lonely and my life no longer mine.

I started being intolerant of everything my poor son did.
I shouted at him if he forgot to close toilet lid!
His homework was confusing; his Grade Seven maths was no mean feat.
I felt incompetent and useless; to my bed I did retreat.

I called upon my friends, as out of bed I could not get.
They took my son to school and back so I could get some rest.
Even though I slept I did not feel that things improved.
Sad and constantly crying, these feelings I could not move.

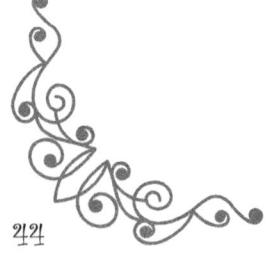

'Why me? Why me?' I asked myself, why did I have that stroke?
These things don't happen to women like me, they happen to unfit folk.
I couldn't see my life get better in any positive way.
So I chatted with my friends online, and my sister rang the doctor that day.

I sat and cried in front of him; I felt a failure sitting there.
All I could talk about was sadness and this feeling of despair.
I recall his words a month ago, it hit me, but perhaps I knew.
"You've got post stroke depression. Don't fight it, let me help you."

So medication was prescribed, something I had not really desired.
But help I needed to balance my brain, even though it would make me tired.
My husband, he took extra leave, to be at home with us.
I didn't have to do a thing, and he didn't make a fuss.

He looked after me so well, despite my teary spells.
He fed me, cared for me, hugged me lots, until I started to feel well.
He went back to work two weeks ago, and I think I'm doing well.
He comes home in two weeks' time, and I'm different, he will tell.

I've penned some poems since my stroke, not all will make you smile.
But I never thought I'd write a poem about this recent awful time.
What I learnt these last few weeks, is that I am not alone.
Depression hits so many of us, without us really knowing.

Once admitted, that's the key, to have the strength to cope.
Don't sit and cry and wonder why, but get up and have some hope.
There are people out there who can help, so maybe let them in,
Instead of sitting on your own and feeling sad within.

Sometimes when I think I want to curl up in my cosy shell,
I look around at what I've got and how I've done so well.
I find it hard being a different 'me' but that is not so bad.
I try to appreciate not what I had but now just what I have.

I've met some lovely people since my stroke, who've helped me through.
The Facebook sites do wondrous things and they can help you too.
'Til my next poem, when I will try to send a happier one your way.
Please don't forget to think of lots of happy thoughts today.

My thoughts, poems and artwork

Everyone you meet is fighting a battle you know nothing about.

*Be kind.
Always.*

Anonymous

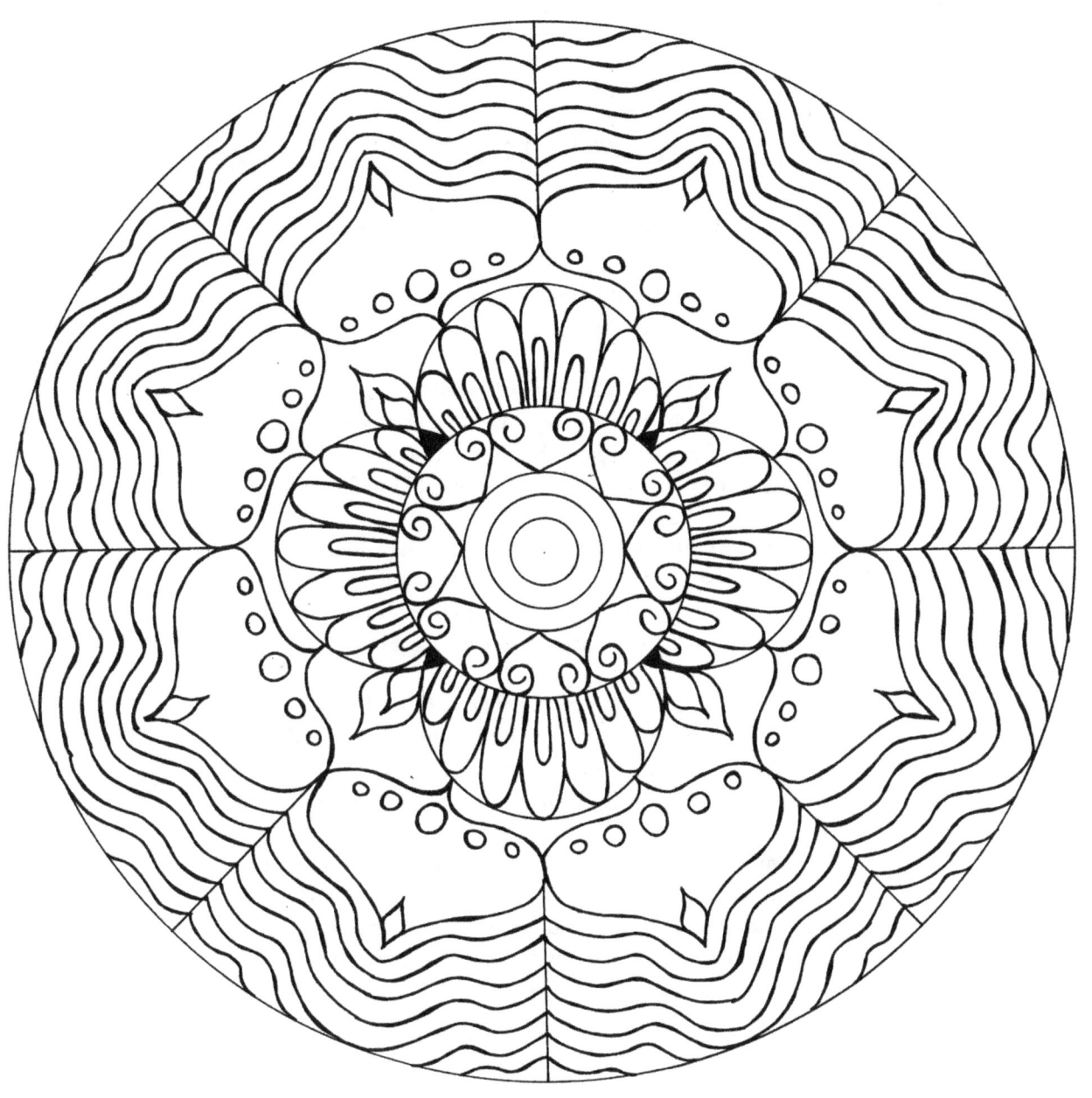

© Sharon Morgan of Manifesting Mandalas
Used with permission.

Muffin maker extraordinaire

I'm bored at home; can't work, can't think.
I'm sick of being tied to the kitchen sink.
My brain won't work like it did before.
Maybe I should do something easy instead of just being bored.

Try some baking, that's what I'll do.
Our soccer club keeps saying "We need mums like you!"
I can't do baking from scratch, don't know where to start.
I could buy some packet muffin mix, or should I make some tarts?

Muffins I think, vanilla and choc chip will be just swell.
Oooh, these are going to be great if they turn out well.
I get the ingredients out and I'm ready to start.
I check, check and check again, have I got every part?

Mixing bowl, scales, jugs and spoons from the larder.
Packet mix, eggs, milk all out on the bench and in order.
I'm ready to start, my excited shout it is so loud.
Am I really going to make muffins? Such a feat, I feel so proud.

I do the vanilla first, in go the eggs, the mix and whisk so frantically.
I follow the instructions and all seems right to me.
The mixture seems a little runny, and I take another look.
I pour it all in the cupcake tins and hope and pray they cook.

Into the oven they all go, a dozen of those cakes.
Now onto the choc chip ones, I'm really feeling great.
I open up my choc chop mix and reach for two eggs to mix.
But where on earth can they now be, I'm in a little fix.

I know I got them from the fridge when I made my other cakes.
I hunt around the kitchen but no eggs are there to take.
And then it hits me, all at once, how silly can I be?
I used four eggs in the vanilla ones, when only two should have been.

And then my milk, I see it there, sitting in the bowl.
I forgot to put the milk in too, I feel like such a fool.
What do I do? Do I give up? No! I soldier on.
I'm in the car, to the shops I go, this battle will be won.

I'm back home in double quick time, my oven's just gone ping.
Those vanilla ones with too many eggs tasted really quite amazing.
I did the choc chip ones right this time and they also came out great.
Then frosting and decorations done and I wasn't even late.

So the moral of this tale my friends, is give anything a go.
You may not be quite up to it and feel a little low.
But everyone likes muffins, with too many eggs or not.
And the soccer boys won't care at all, they'll no doubt scoff the lot!

*Life is like a camera.
Just focus on what's important,
capture the good times,
develop from the negatives
and if things don't work out,
just take another shot.*

Author unknown

Down day

Today's not good, I don't know why.
I seem to want to sit and cry.
But why today, why can it be?
What's changed in me, please can you see?

I don't understand why I have these days.
When I cannot think, nor do, just laze.
Days like today, I don't want them to stay.
So I try to will these feelings away.

But they won't go; I don't know what to do.
Ring a friend? Take a walk? Do something new?
To bed, quite often I must go.
And sleep off my feelings so they don't show.

I know I'm lucky, I can do that in a shot.
I have no little ones who needs their mum and all she has got.
But when school's out, I get myself right.
As I still have a son who needs me tonight.

It's homework, then dinner and cuddles some nights.
I know that tomorrow I will be alright.
And bed, here it comes, where I've spent all my day,
where I hope that this desperate feeling will at last go away.

Thankfully these down days are rarer as the months progress.
And getting through them each time, it just means having rest.
I know we can't all rest as families take our time.
But all I know rest is the key, and I will soon be feeling fine.

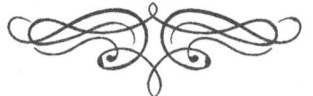

I may not be there yet, but I'm closer than I was yesterday.

Author unknown

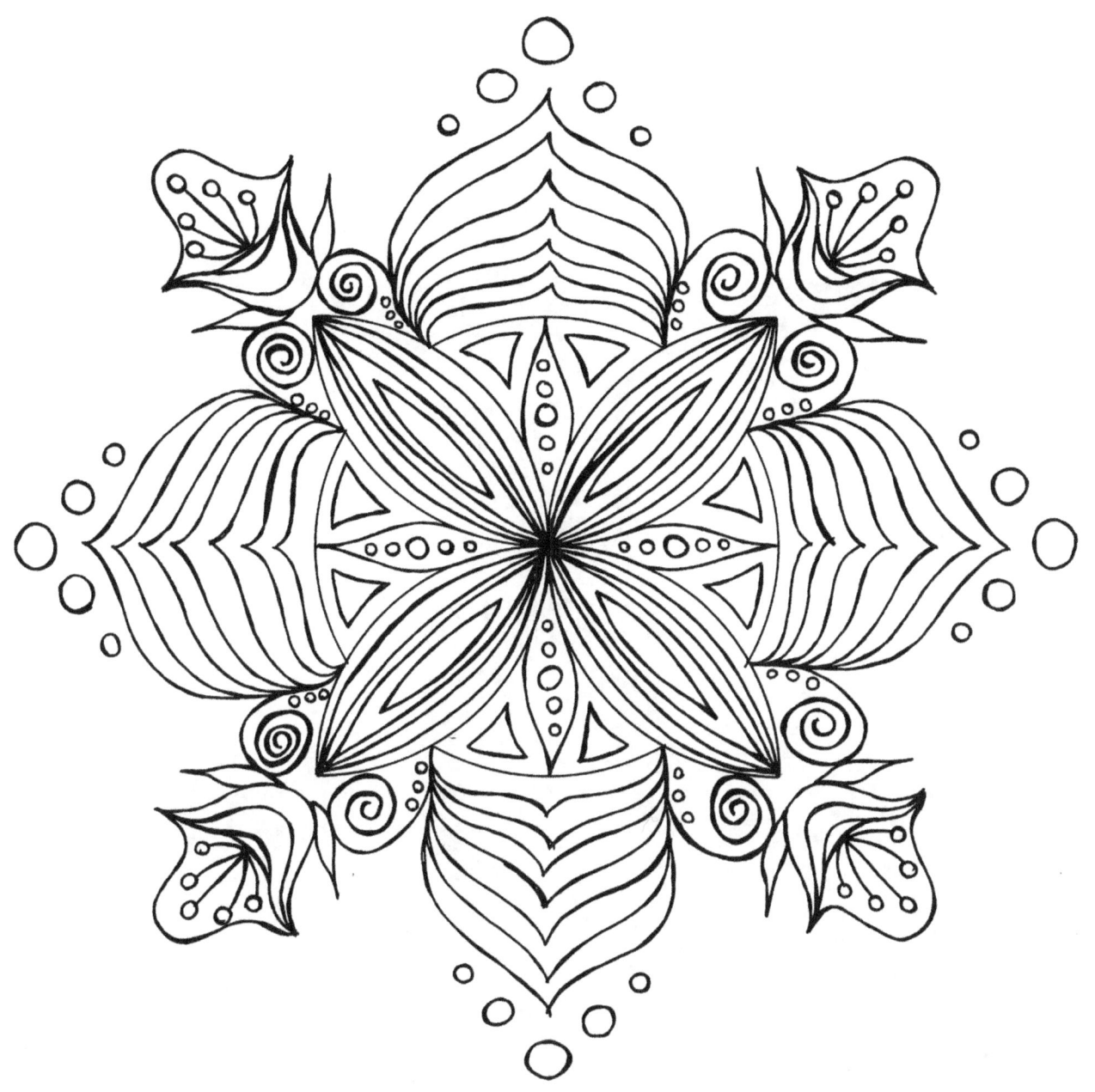

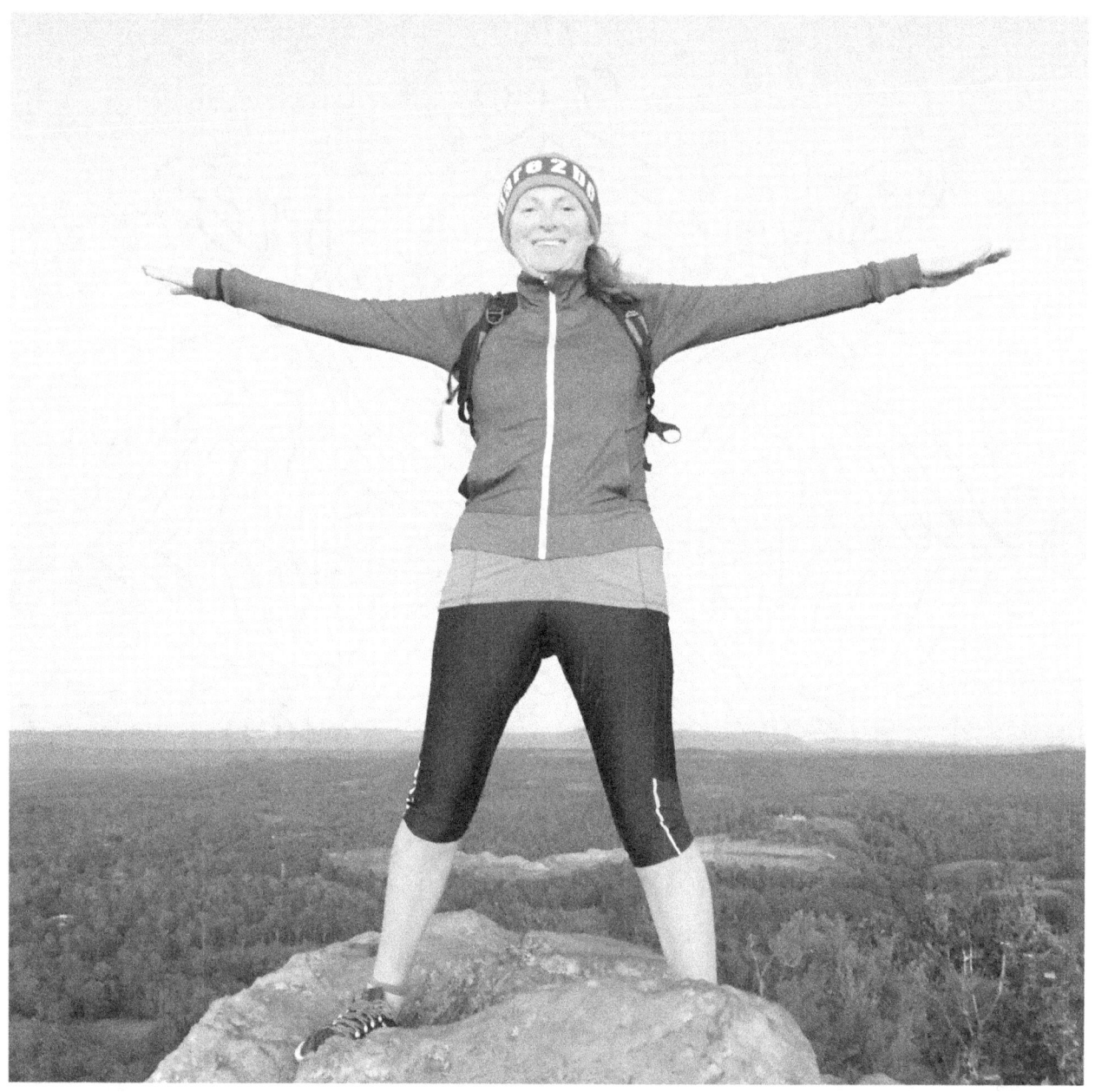

I want to climb a mountain

I want to climb a mountain, but I'm no longer fit.
I want to climb a mountain, Mount Ngungun will be it.
But how does one climb a mountain? I've not done it before.
I get so tired just from walking, and lie shattered on the floor.

But I *can* climb a mountain, I know that if I try,
and get myself all fit again, then who is to reason why?
I know I'll climb a mountain, but maybe not today.
My friends are having coffee, and sitting by the bay.

I'll climb it maybe next week, or two months after that.
When I know I will get to the top and be very proud of that.
If you want to climb a mountain, please just let me know,
then we can get together and organise a day to go.

Maybe I'll go to Victoria and climb one they have there.
I'd celebrate with friends at the top, a hug then we can share.
Or maybe go to St. Louis, and see a friend half way down.
I'm sure that will be heaps of fun and together we can clown around.

Perhaps I'll climb it in Austin, with another friend by my side.
We can count our eggs for muffins, and be sure they're all inside.
Wherever I climb a mountain, I will do it one day soon.
And then maybe I'll do something else - perhaps fly to the moon?

Feeling low

Today I'm feeling low.
There's just no place to go.
Please let me go and hide,
as I feel so sad inside.

Stop telling me I'll soon be well.
Not one of you can really tell
how much I hurt today.
Please will you all go away.

This feeling that I have.
It's not good, it feels so bad.
The desperation in my voice,
somehow I know it is my choice.

I hope it doesn't last.
I thought this feeling would be past.
But each day it gets much worse.
Will I end up in a hearse?

I don't really want to die.
I just want to shut my eyes and fly.
So the pain can go away
and I won't feel as bad today.

But that feeling never comes.
And my head, it sort of hums
with feelings of despair
And what's happening out there.

I know you love me so.
I hope you understand and go.
My rest it is the key.
Even if I wallow in self-pity.

So today I choose to rest
and hope tomorrow is my best.
But if tomorrow isn't grand,
then leave me be, please understand.

*Don't forget you're human.
It's okay to have a meltdown.
Just don't unpack
and live there.
Cry it out and then focus on
where you are headed.*

Anonymous

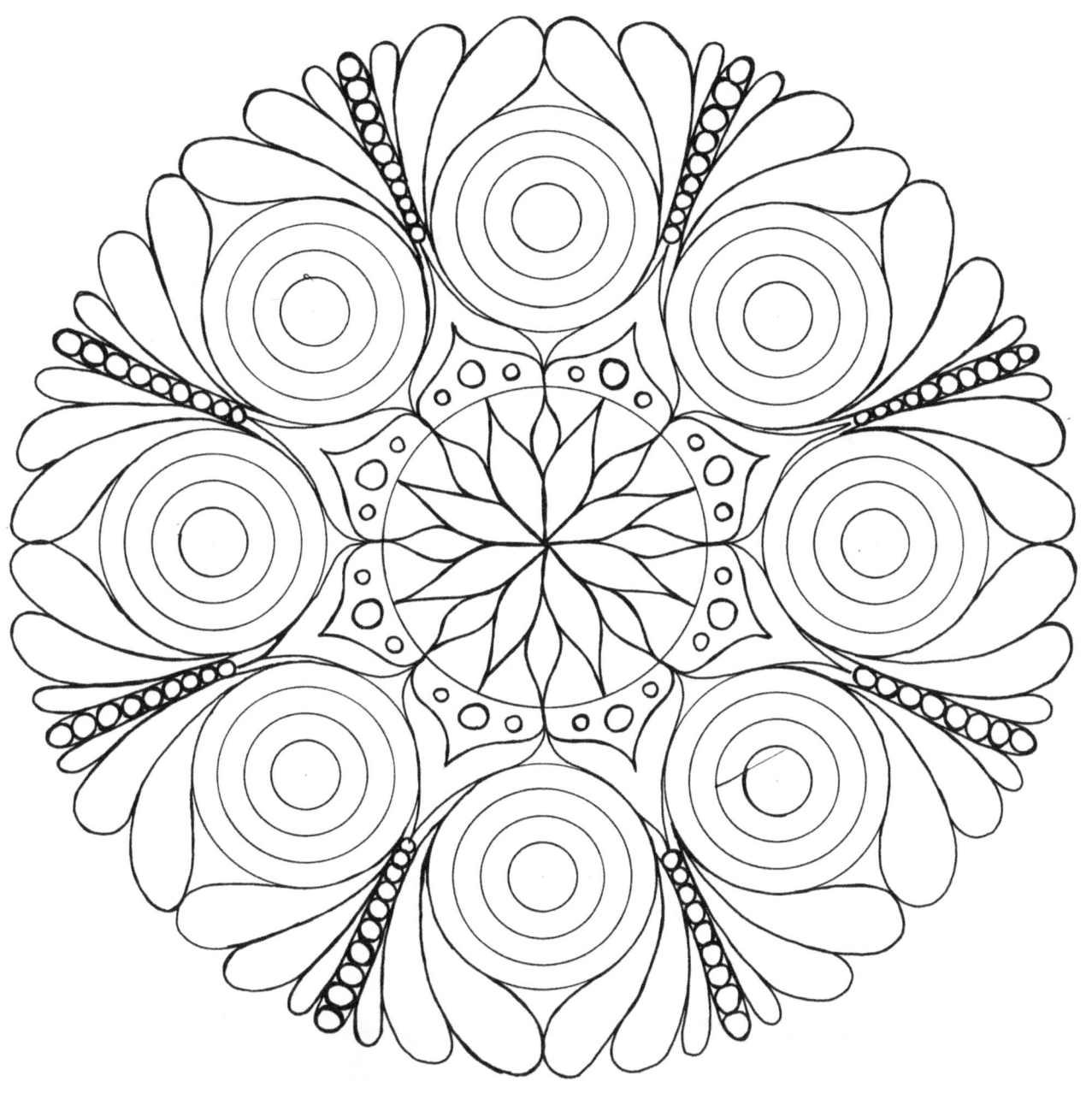

© Sharon Morgan of Manifesting Mandalas
Used with permission.

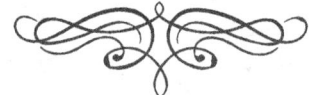

*People inspire you,
or they drain you.
Pick them wisely.*

Hans F. Hansen

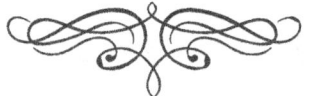

Financial advisor phobia

Today is the day he visited, the financial advisor man.
With his knowledge, facts and figures of things I don't understand.
My husband, lovely David, he says it will be okay.
I need not worry about anything, just listen what he has to say.

I have my notepad ready, plus my trusty pen.
And off he goes with gobbledygook, what is it with these men?
Am I supposed to understand these terms? They mean nothing to me.
And then I look at David who looks busy drinking tea.

I'll make some notes then, I thought it best.
I felt I was being put to the test.
Super, pensions, on and on he droned.
My goodness, when will this man go home?

An hour later, my brain so full, he left.
I sighed and sobbed, at last my brain can rest.
"I'll leave it with you," he said with glee.
Was he saying that seriously?

My notes I took, I could not read.
How the heck am I supposed to know what we need?
"Forget it all," my husband said.
"We'll talk about it later, before we go to bed."

But I'm a perfectionist, or at least I was.
My notes need to make sense, this was my job.
So I typed and deciphered and made them neat.
The figures and the words were at last complete.

We didn't talk it through that night, that's for another time.
Who wants to talk about pensions when I could be drinking wine!

I wish I had wings

As I lie in my bed and look up to the sky,
I wish I had feathery wings so I could try to fly.

I'd find a fluffy white cloud, and sit there all day long.
I'd say "Hi" to the birds as they flew by, and listen to their songs.

I'd wait till it rained, and watch the ground below.
And see all the trees and flowers as they then started to grow.

I'd see the people and the animals, rushing all around,
bumping into each other, as they hurry across the ground.

As the breeze comes through my window, and flutters on my head,
I really wish that I could fly, instead of being in bed.

I seem to do so well, for days, and weeks at my best.
My energy gets better and I seem to need less rest.

My limits, I thought I knew them, so I carry on as I do.
But then one day it hits me, and my head explodes to goo.

I find it so frustrating, not being the normal me.
I can hear everyone saying "Just be patient, you will see".

But I don't want to be patient; I want to be like everyone.
I want to climb mountains, and have a lot of fun.

I had fun at the weekend, with good friends and family.
I've maybe overdone it, and now this week is rest for me.

My head, it won't stop pounding, the meds they are increased.
I'm totally good for nothing; all I want right now is peace.

So please, dear God, just help me, and teach me what is 'slow'.
As I really can't take more of this, as everyone will know.

Thank goodness I've got friends around and family close to me.
And Lilly always right by my side, as cuddly as can be.

My son, he is tremendous, he looks after me when I'm bad.
But it's not fair, it shouldn't be like this, he is such a grown up lad.

So Santa, when you leave the North Pole on Christmas Eve this year,
please put some wings inside your sack and leave them for me here.

And when it gets too much for me, I'll put them on and fly,
instead of staying in my bed, and having to explain why.

I'll maybe take my boy along, with his iPad, there's no doubt.
And maybe for only one day, we'll shut the whole world out.

'Til then, my bed will have to do, as I suppose it helps me rest.
A few hours hence, my husband's home, I will be feeling at my best.

Maybe I can still dream of wings, if it helps to get me right.
And hope and pray that maybe once, I'll have a good sleep tonight.

No matter how you feel…
Get up
Dress up
Show up

Regina Brett

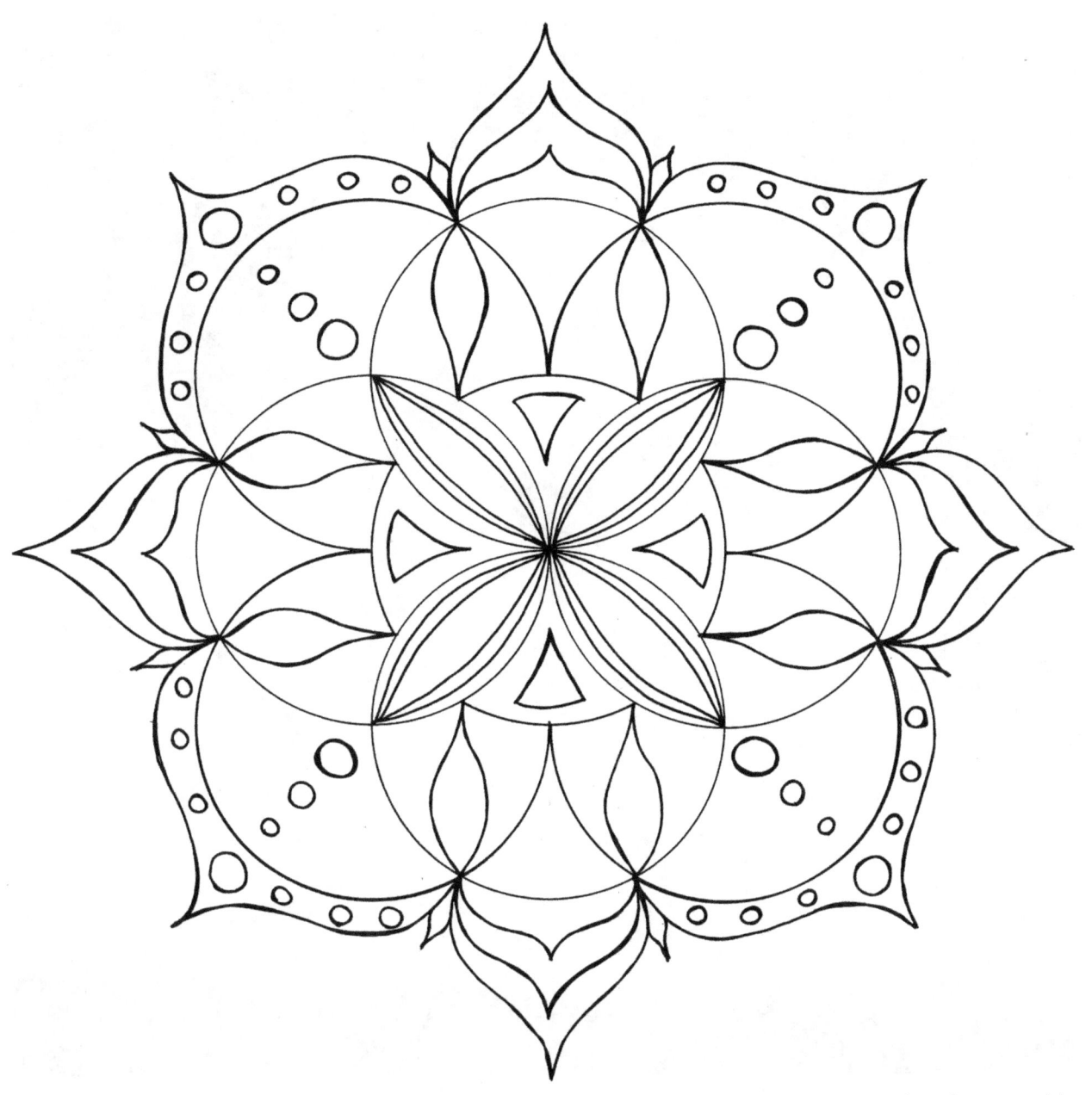

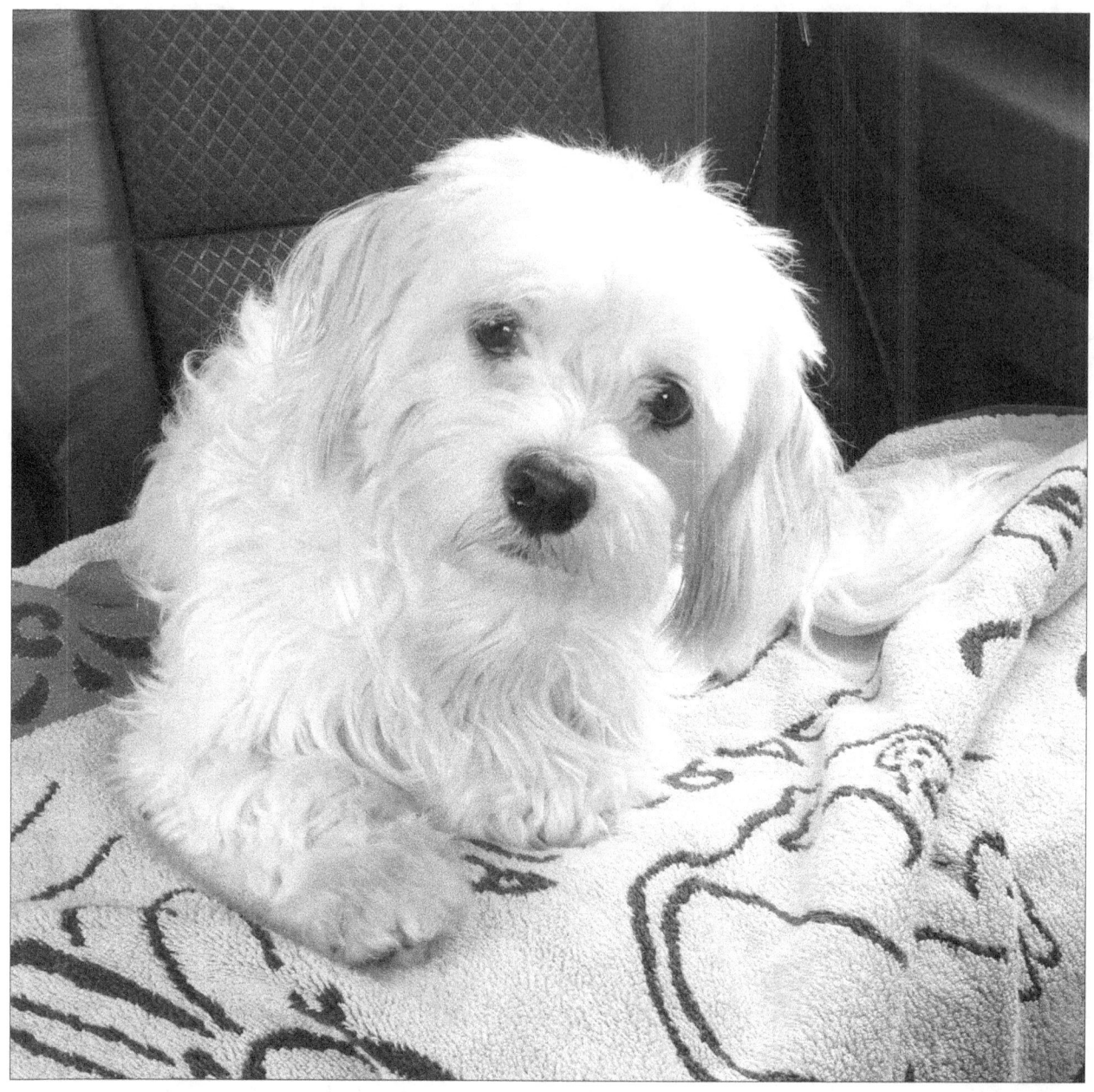

Our Lilly

We got our lovely Lilly five months ago today.
We got her from the refuge, but she hadn't been a stray.
She lived with an old lady, who got sick and then she died.
And poor fluffy little Lilly was so desperate inside.

She fretted and she worried and she got a skin disease.
In quarantine for five weeks, until she felt at ease.
Her skin cleared up a little, but she wasn't still 'for sale',
until she'd tried some special food and grew fur on her tail.

The day we went to visit, was a day that changed for me.
She looked at us with those sad eyes, and ours she had to be.
We took her within half an hour, with her rash and food and all.
And went straight home to settle her, 'Our Lilly' was ours to call.

She didn't play, she didn't bark, she did not do much at all.
She didn't even know how to fetch and bring us back a ball.
She sat with me before my stroke, only me, and not my lad.
So when I was in hospital, she fretted and was sad.

When I came home from hospital, I saw Our Lilly and I cried.
Poor Lilly must have thought that her new owner had also died.
The welcoming, the barking and the sitting on my knee,
helped me get back up again and aided my recovery.

Now five months on, Our Lilly has changed so drastically.
She barks, she plays and goes for walks and now, not just with me.
I love her so, and even now, as I sit and pen this poem,
she's sat right by the side of me, a lapdog of my own.

Six months on

Six months on, where should I be?
I don't think I shall ever again feel like 'me'.
A stroke changed my life on that fateful day
and I still don't like how I feel this way.

I always seem tired in my body and my head,
and the only relief is to spend time in bed.
I used to be fit and bags of energy I had.
Now when I walk any distance, it makes me feel so bad.

The days seem so long, I can't wait for them to end.
Doing nothing much at all almost sends me round the bend!
I used to feel jolly and really happy all the time.
Now to just get through each day is what's always on my mind.

My husband, he is home now, support he can give.
But what I hope and pray for, is once again to 'live'.
I feel my life has little meaning, which I know is so bad.
This feeling I have sometimes, well it just makes me so sad.

I know all my friends on the FAST parenting site, they will know.
And someone please tell me how to let these feelings go.
I know many of you suffered strokes a long, long time ago,
but these feelings I have, clearly take a while to go.

Maybe I'm rushing it? Am I expecting too much?
I no longer believe I have the Midas touch.
I've rarely wondered 'why me?' but today I do.
Maybe tomorrow will be better. Who am I kidding, me or you?

As I sit and pen this poem and my husband sits with me,
the sun is shining brightly, so what cares should there really be?
He is my rock, my friend, my lover (we shall get to that real soon).
I couldn't think of anyone else to share a sunny afternoon.

My son is doing well at school, these months he's grown up fast.
I'm really quite surprised to think how these six have passed.
I try to think of positive things, since I had my stroke
And one of them for definite, is meeting lots of lovely folk.

Instead of drowning in self-pity, I should stop thinking about what I had.
Stop dreaming about what is gone, as this new life ain't so bad.
So off to bed I go now, and a nanny nap to have.
I am sure that by tomorrow, I will not feel half as bad.

It's only oranges

It's Saturday tomorrow, well that's come around quite quick.
Who will they be playing this week, let's take your pick.
Where are we going, what time to be there?
I wonder if it will be somewhere I can take my chair?

To ask my son, there's no point in that.
He rarely remembers his soccer hat.
So it's down to Mum, the answers to seek
As Dad is still away working, now in his fourth week.

The timetable I put on the fridge for both of us to see.
An early game I see it is, no lie in then, for me.
So up we get, its 7am, is this necessary?
Saturdays should be lazy days, especially for me.

A cuppa made, too early for food, and off we jolly well go.
But halfway along the journey, realise no soccer boots in tow.
A row, a fall out, "It's not my fault" he tries to plead with me.
"It's too early to be getting up" he says so earnestly.

We go back home, and dash straight in, the car door left ajar.
The dog thinks we've come back for her and gets into the car.
The dog settled back into the house, we leave, but now he's glum.
I know he doesn't like it when I'm an angry, shouting mum.

We get to the ground, nowhere to park, with chair and flask we run.
I think I'm going to vomit or at least end up on my bum.
I find a spot, say hello to all and sit down on my chair.
"The half time fruit?" I am then asked and respond in despair.

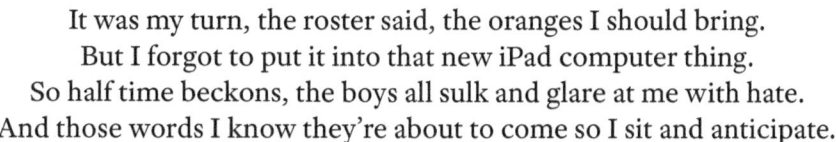

It was my turn, the roster said, the oranges I should bring.
But I forgot to put it into that new iPad computer thing.
So half time beckons, the boys all sulk and glare at me with hate.
And those words I know they're about to come so I sit and anticipate.

"No oranges! How can that be? How could she be so lax?"
I fiddle and squirm inside my chair and wish they'd cut me some slack.
The second half ends, the game is won, I gather up my things.
But the travel home is now with sadness, for oranges I did not bring.

I feel so bad about my plight but next week is far away.
No oranges to think about now, on this lovely sunny day.
We go straight home, the dog goes mad with happiness we are there.
And then comes Patrick, hugs me lots and I hope he doesn't care.

He tells me that it doesn't matter, and forgiving as he is.
"It's silly Mum, its only oranges" and then gives me a kiss.
About the oranges, who gives a hoot, the fact they won is best.
"But Mum, you know next week it is your turn to take the vests?"

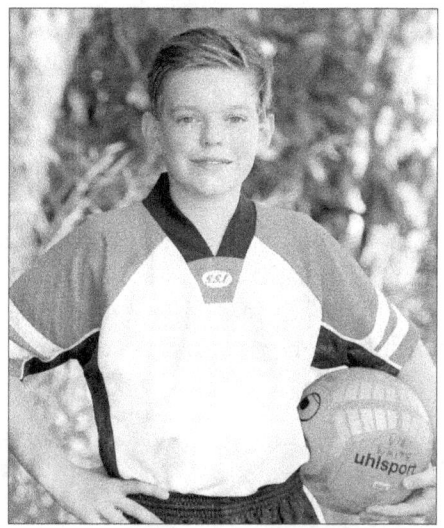

Non-working mum

This week, it has been tiring, with lots and lots to do.
I've sorted cupboards and drawers galore and fixed up Patrick's loo.
To think this time last August, as much as I recall,
I'd many big investigations, charted on my office wall.

A cop I was a few years ago, left in 2008.
And five years here in Australia, a Private Investigator I did make.
My life has changed dramatically, I'm sure you all will know.
Now what's important to me now, is how my life will go.

A busy working mum I was, well, not too busy to be true.
I still had time for fun and games and oft a drink or two.
But since my stroke, my days have changed, oh what am I to do?
I feel okay most of the time, but my brain is full of goo.

I need to make so many lists, my iPad stores the lot.
And if it is not on the list, I will forget it in a jot.
Multi-tasking, what a laugh, a 'man brain' now I have.
If things don't get done one at a time, I stress and that is that!

My brain has changed so much; I was such an organised girl.
But now, I find my thoughts are always in such a silly whirl.
I'm walking now with friends some days, but not as often as before.
Too much walking makes me tired and I'm asleep by half past four!

I write my poems, as you all know, to keep my brain occupied.
And most days, no matter what I do, my brain is really tired.
Some cabinets, they are still closed, that's what the doctors say.
And maybe, possibly, they'll open one eventful day.

But perhaps I need new thoughts, I ponder to myself.
Maybe it is time now, for some new books on the shelf.
As I type this, I sit outside, Lilly dog on my knee.
It makes me finally realise the person I could be.

Just because I do not work, that's okay, I can do something else.
My stroke has taught me to embrace parts of my inner self.
I'm a good mum, wife and friend and that's what life is all about.
Even if these roles may lapse when tiredness wins out.

Perhaps it's not about working, but what I'm trying to say.
If I feel good about what I've done, then that's another positive day.
So do your best, that's all there is, don't beat yourself up too.
Your family will understand as you know that they love you.

My thoughts, poems and artwork

*It's not WHAT
I have in my life
but WHO I have in
my life that counts.*

Nishan Panwar

The party animal no more

I used to love to go out socialising with friends and family.
But nowadays, the evenings are somewhat of a chore for me.
I have to rest before I go, or I'm shot by half past eight.
Forget it if you want me to drink as well as stay up late.

I love my food and like a drink, but not in the same vein as before.
If I try you'd have to pick me up from the restaurant floor.
The noise and chatter are just too much; I just don't stand a chance.
And as for any live music, well please don't expect me to dance.

When I get tired, my slurring starts, it's not too good to hear.
Then a burning sensation starts in my face that goes from ear to ear.
It starts off in my ears, moves to my cheeks and flows into my head.
The throbbing, burning pain I feel; I just need to go to bed.

The brain ache, well, it then takes hold; I can't stop it, although I try.
I have to excuse myself right then and there before I start to cry.
My friends, they know me now so well and do not despair with me.
Our get-togethers suit my tired brain, they are as quiet as can be.

The places we go, where there is little noise,
They help me so immensely, and I'm grateful for choice.
A party animal I once was, but for now I'll take it slow.
There are plenty of quiet places to choose for me to go.

So the evenings, they're spent mainly home, cuddling with my son.
Now, is that such a hardship, or am I a lucky mum?

The luckiest wife in the world

My husband David Brennand, now what does he portray?
He's loving, caring, funny, and smart, "Not bad" I hear you say.
I met him 17 years ago, it doesn't seem that long.
The years have flown he will agree, he would say he does no wrong.

A blind date was set up for us, in a restaurant close to home.
Arranged by friends who knew we should no longer be alone.
The night was good, nice he seemed, and he had some things to say.
Other dates followed and two years on, we had our wedding day.

Some diamond earrings he designed and gave to me with pride.
I knew he was the man for me, as I stood wearing them at his side.
We had some fun, took holidays and enjoyed our time together.
We both knew that a family would make our lives much better.

So the next year from our wedding day, our son Patrick arrived.
That changed our lives so drastically, my goodness, we were tired.
David changed into a different man and new qualities came out.
A doting father for all these years, of that there is no doubt.

He's nurtured, taught, and loved our son, these past 13 years.
He's seen from us such fun and laughs and perhaps even some tears.
Our move to Oz, which changed our lives, for the better of us all.
And supported all our concerns and doubts and we have had a ball.

I had a stroke now nine months ago and I know that hit him bad.
He thought he'd lost me on that horrid day; I know it makes him sad.
He's got me through, as times before, he makes me forget my woes.
His humour and his loving ways make me stronger as each day goes.

He worked away for several months, a month at a time it was.
But then the contract ended and he was back at home with us.
This last month has been marvellous, he's not sat on his bum.
He's worked his little socks off and we've had a bit of fun.

I now have three new toilets, a challenge I know for him.
When he returns in three weeks, there'll be sinks for him to put in!
He's done the shopping, cooking and more, but now today he left.
A new contract starts, another year away, but no more than three weeks' away at best.

Patrick, Lilly and I will cope again, as we always do.
He worries and frets for us when he's away, but he really shouldn't do.
We've lots of friends who lend a hand and a sister who helps me too.
My energy levels have improved and my brain's not as full of goo!

I know he'll be embarrassed, when he knows I've written this.
But I wanted all the world to know what a fantastic man he is.
He is my rock, without a doubt, for that is oh so true.
And I love him now with all my heart, as I always do.

*Happiness isn't about
getting what you want
all the time;
it's about loving
what you have.*

Asher Roth

School holidays

School holidays will soon be here. I'm stressed and they've not begun!
No more lazing round the house, my son will need some fun.
I've play days to sort and parks and beach, so many things to do.
More muffins (oh no!) to make for parties, and a visit to the zoo.

I can't cope with it; my brain's too full of what to do each day.
Please can the school holidays just come and go straight away?
As usual, I've friends on hand, to help me through this time.
They'll organise just where to go, what to bring and where we dine.

The inflatables, they're always good, just go to the pool and sit.
And watch him falling in the water, no stress, not even a bit.
The beach nearby, now that's great fun, I sit and watch him play.
I can have a coffee and relax, so why am I stressing this way?

I just don't know, I should snap out of it, there really is no worry.
We'll take each day one at a time, and nothing in a hurry.
Patrick loves to read, thank goodness for that, so quiet times there are.
And if some days I don't feel so good, we don't have to go too far.

So bring them on, these holidays, and more challenges ahead.
And once they've gone I shall resume my life back in my bed!

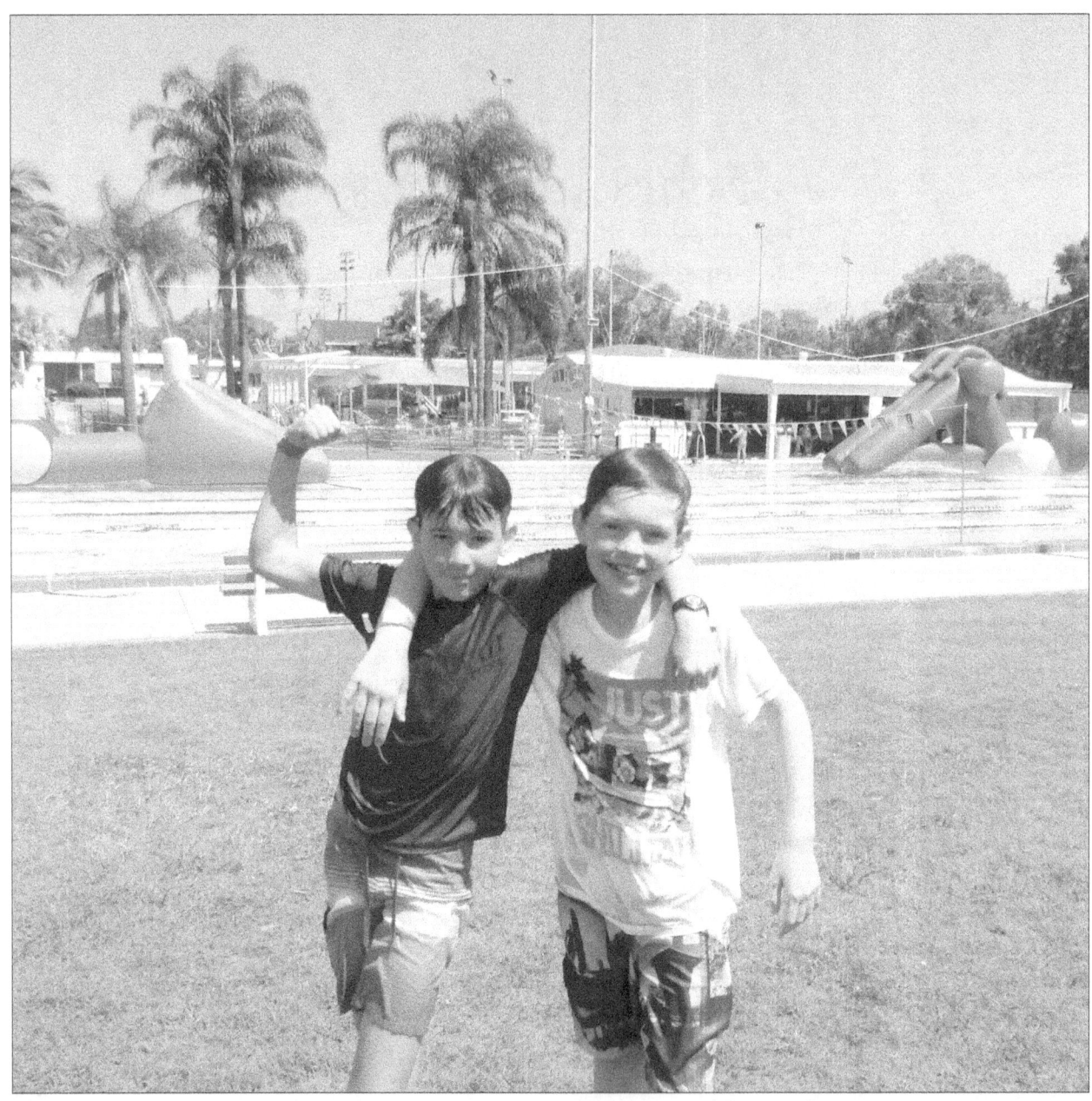

The inflatables

I'm sitting here at the local swimming pool, with Patrick and his mate.
Two best friends together in the pool, now what is there to hate?
They both love the inflatables, they often tell me so.
I think when it ends in two hours' time, they will not want to go.

I love to watch them playing, getting wet and wild.
They climb to the very top, then throw each other down the slide.
They sometimes like to sit on top, but the staff won't let them stay.
Out comes the dreaded hosepipe and water splashes them both away.

There are so many kids today, the sun is shining bright.
They're all running, laughing, screaming, with such a great delight.
I love to watch the kids at play, having so much fun.
Happily I've found a shady tree so I'm cool out in the sun.

I've got my water, iPad and my favourite chair, so I'm organised today.
I can simply sit and watch the boys and everyone else at play.
We'll stay for lunch; well, hot chips no doubt it will be.
Not very healthy, but a naughty treat for them and maybe me.

Maybe an ice cream later on, before Mitchell has to go home.
The late afternoon spent with Patrick and I, once more on our own.

As I look around, and see what else is going on.
I'm listening to the music, it's a very happy song.
I don't want to be anywhere else just now, I am feeling just fine.
Maybe join me next week when we will come another time?

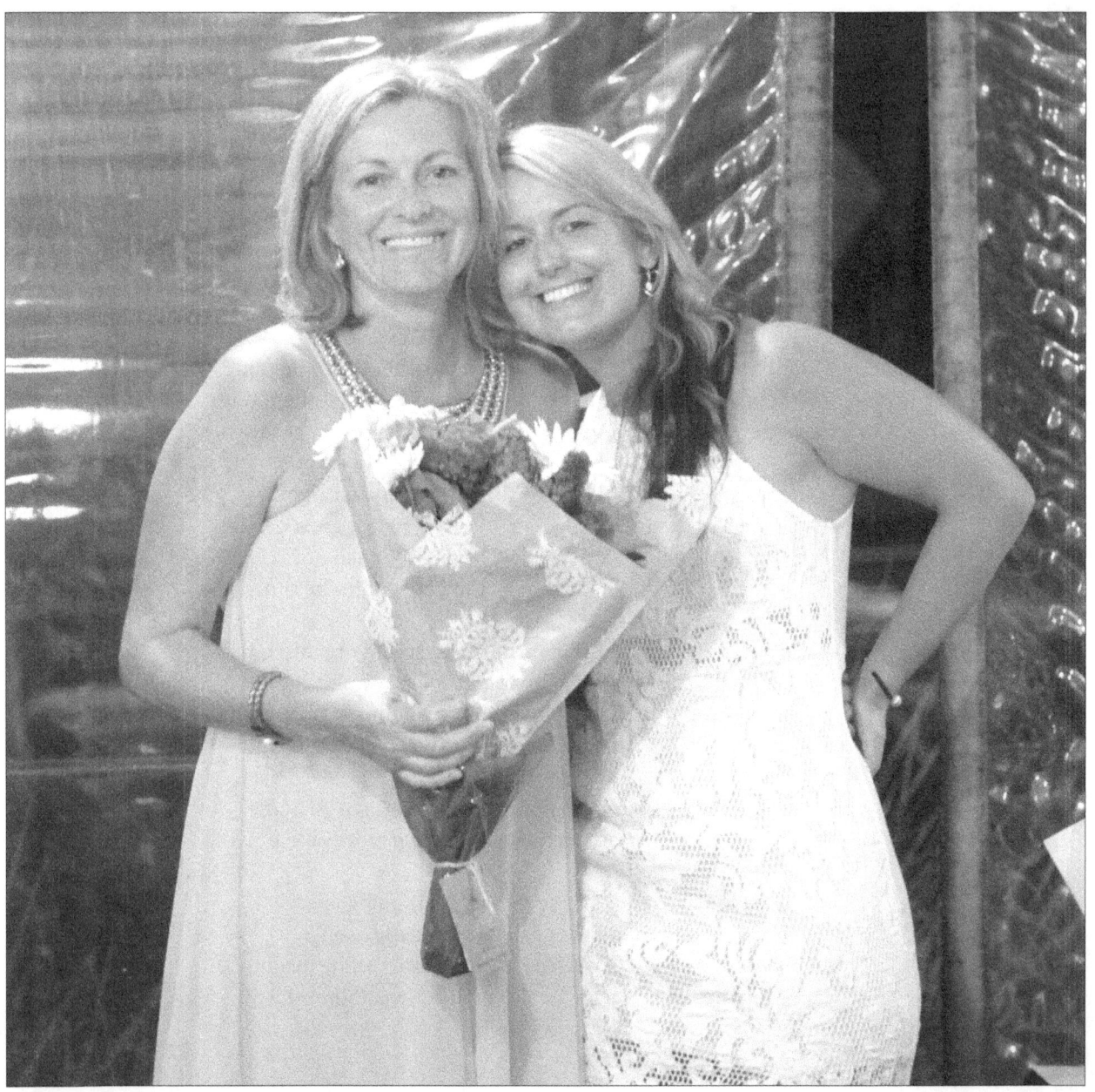

End of challenge thankyou

As I sit here at the end of challenge dinner,
because it has sadly come to an end.
I contemplate my ten week journey
surrounded with lovely new friends.

The challenges, well they have been awesome,
whether I came first or often last.
The main theme about all the adventures
is fitness, teamwork and to have a good blast!

Some of us lost that goal weight,
a tremendous effort for all that we've done.
And others they now are more mind-fit,
and are still struggling with the perfect flat tum!

What I'm saying is it really doesn't matter,
the reasons we signed up for this.
As long as we are better people,
and love our body for now what it is.

So what to do now that it's over?
Will I train as hard as I've done?
The importance I know is to eat cleanly,
and keep training, but make fitness fun!

Oh...before I end this little ditty,
I should acknowledge those who brought me to here.
The three amazing trainers I had,
to support me when I shed a tear.

So thank you all from one grateful challenger,
even though at times you've had to shout.
You are so immensely hard working and awesome,
and deserve this accolade without a doubt.

Life is 10 percent what you make it, and 90 percent how you take it.

Irving Berlin

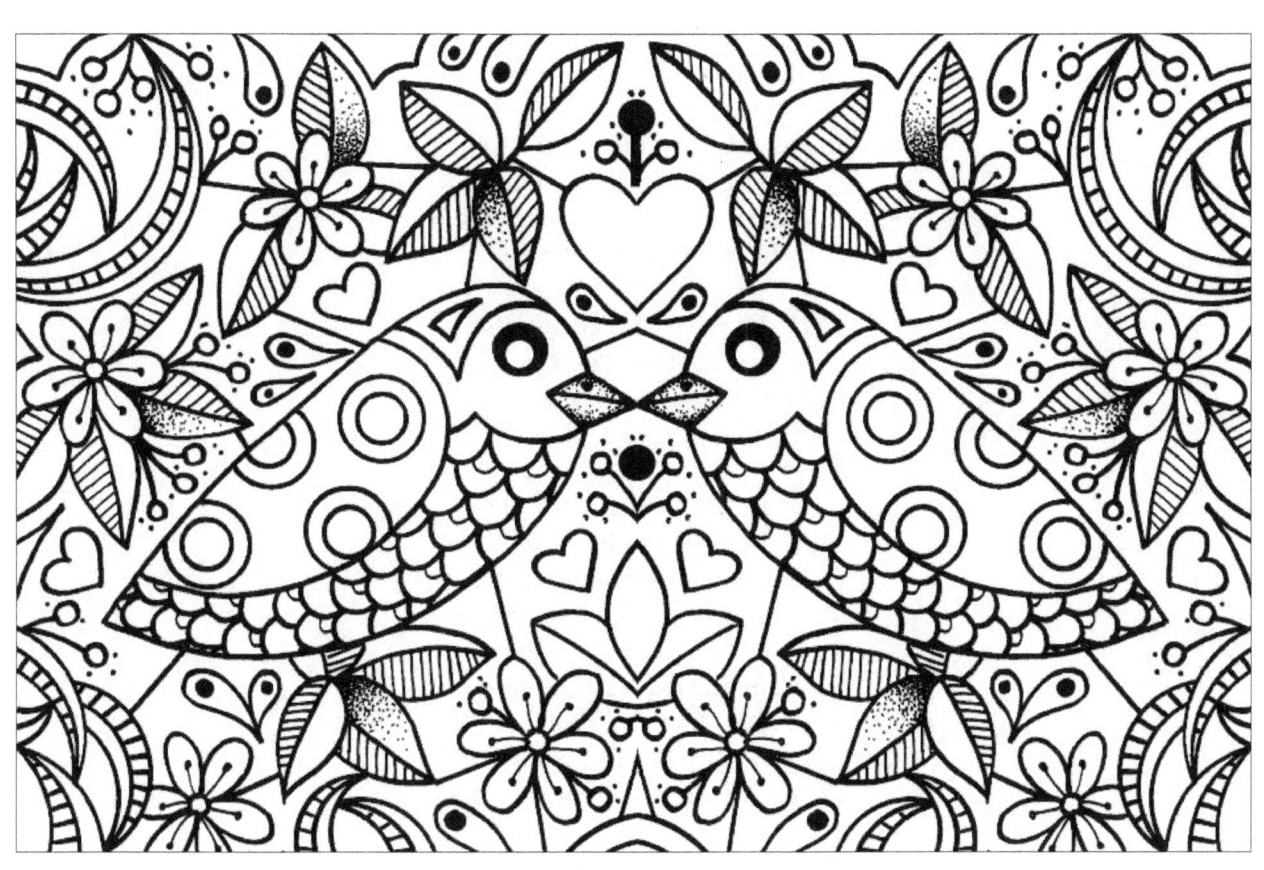

Climbing mountains now

Today we climbed a mountain.
Mt Beerburrum was the one.
We all got there for 8am
and thought we'd have some fun.

Then the trainer brought out the wooden logs.
What were we all to do?
To climb the mountains holding logs
in lots of groups of two!

As if this wasn't a challenge itself,
this mountain, 280m high.
We all looked much less happy
I think some wanted to cry!

No arms to help us push along
those weary bodies of ours.
Few smiles were on our faces
as we stood there by our cars.

So what did we girls do?
Did we cry and all bail out?
NO! We picked up the logs and off we went.
We'd reach the top, there was no doubt.

Once at the top, after a steep incline,
we managed to get some rest.
After snack, a photo and a little dance,
we were again feeling our best.

Then the words "Shall we do it again?"
were uttered by someone.
"Why not?" we all exclaimed with glee,
"It can't be as hard as the first one."

The second time up to the top,
it really was so tough.
But we all did it, how good is that?
But twice was just enough!

Now 560 metres are clocked
for those who were counting their climbs.
There's two weeks left to carry on.
Time to do it again several times.

We are all doing amazing
so please remember this.
And if you haven't started yet,
there's no need to be in a tizz.

Do any mountain, when you can
when you're free of work and home.
And let us know just where and when,
so you won't have to climb alone.

*Fitness is not about being better
than someone else…
it's about being better
than you used to be.*

Brett Hoebel

I did it!

When we first came to Australia,
seven years ago this year.
Our Lady of Rosary was Patrick's school.
Many memories we still hold dear.

Each year they organise a fundraiser
held here on the Coast.
The Caloundra Foreshore Fun Run it is,
and well attended by most.

There's a 10K, 5K and so much more,
a beautiful family day.
You can even take a 3K walk
and participate that way.

So, the first year I attended
I did the 3K walk.
Run? No chance. You're having a laugh.
I'd much rather walk and talk.

As the years progressed
and I saw those runners coming through.
I thought "Maybe, am I serious?
Is that something I could do?"

I'd watched my good friends running
and some had suffered a stroke like me.
They'd trained and got so fit again.
That's where I aspired to be.

Even after my stroke recovery
and getting fitter by the day.
Without the correct training
a 10K run? There was no way.

My friend suggested a personal trainer
based here on the Coast.
If I joined their runners' eight week plan
maybe a 10K I could then boast.

So, with my personal trainer,
and boot camps through the week.
I added on the running course.
I tell you, it was no mean feat!

Many mornings up at 5am.
Is that really a time to rise?
Some training sessions were really tough.
The trainers I grew to despise!

I hurt my knee on a training run.
That really set me back.
Physiotherapy sorted that out,
and the day came around real fast.

I was feeling very nervous
But my mind set got me through.
If I was going to achieve this goal of mine,
I knew what I had to do.

As I ran downhill to Moffat Beach,
the finish line in my view.
I saw my son waiting to run with me.
Tears welled and then I knew.

I've really gone and done it!
I've actually run 10K.
A goal I thought I would never reach
I well achieved that day.

Ding-a-lingin'

When I started fitness training,
now over a year and a half ago.
I tried some things I'd never done
and did every one with great gusto.

At the same time I started cycling
with friends here on the Coast.
I'd always had a bicycle
but not ridden it much, like most.

Those Wednesdays came a calling,
with friends I'd got to know.
We cycled along the headland.
There were us three girls in tow.

We often cycled 20k's,
always the coastal path.
Each Wednesday we'd meet up at Bill's.
We always had a laugh.

Then my husband's contract ended
and home to us he came.
"Can I come out with you three girls?"
One day he did exclaim.

So, 'Dave and the Ding-a-Lings' were formed
On one sunny Wednesday morn'.
Even though he didn't have a bell
it didn't matter at all.

My sister then, she joined us
and many more have added on.
We now have quite a gathering
as we cycle through the sun.

So if you are free on Wednesdays,
why don't you give one of us a call?
We promise to take it gently
and I guarantee you'll have a ball.

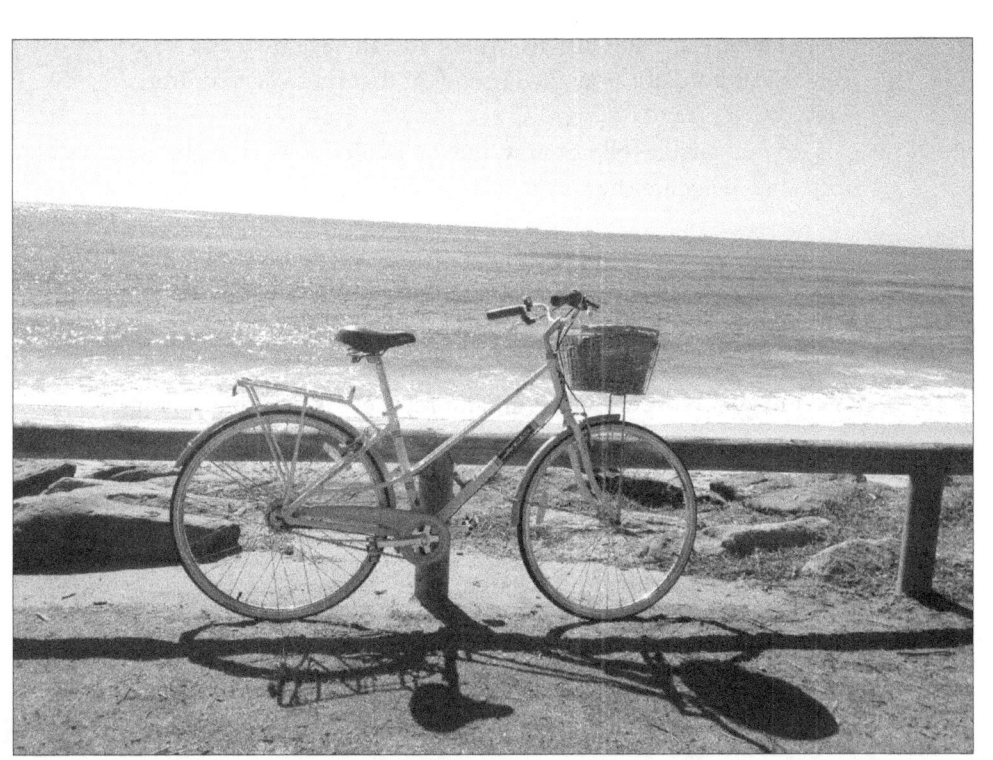

Happy, two years on

Where am I now? What do I do?
Is my life good now? Is my brain still full of goo?

I still pinch myself, to think it's now two years ago,
when my darling son found me on that cold, tiled bathroom floor.

I've had my ups and downs, which you all have read about.
But as I sit here now, my life is good, of that there is no doubt.

I do not work, well not now, maybe I will not ever again.
But I love my life the way it is, never looking back to 'then'.

I love my fitness through the week; sometimes David joins me too.
We walk the dog, we cycle and we run a kilometre or two.

I spend more time with Patrick, always taking him here and there.
With volleyball, soccer, scouts and more, there is no time to spare.

I have a little craft room where I make greetings cards for friends.
I often wonder where the day has gone, when it comes to an end.

I think about my life back then, a busy working mum.
I no longer wish I had it back, these days, it is more fun.

I have more time for important things, my family for one.
These things we perhaps didn't focus on when work had to be done.

I don't regret the fact that I had my stroke that fateful day.
I really feel it was meant to be, God telling me in his own way.

To take a slower pace in life, don't stress, don't do too much.
We all should take heed before we all get that stressed out touch!

So as I now have passed my two years, and see how far I've come.
It's time to celebrate my life, and my achievements that I've done.

Without my stroke, my book would not have been written for you all.
That in itself is amazing, and believe me, I've had a ball.

A little hard to get to print, but got there in the end.
So many people to thank for this, my gratitude I send.

I hope you've enjoyed my poetry, the funny and sad times too.
Please look after yourself, be healthy, be fit and thanks to all of you.

"What day is it?"
"It's today," squeaked Piglet.
"My favourite day," said Pooh.

A.A. Milne

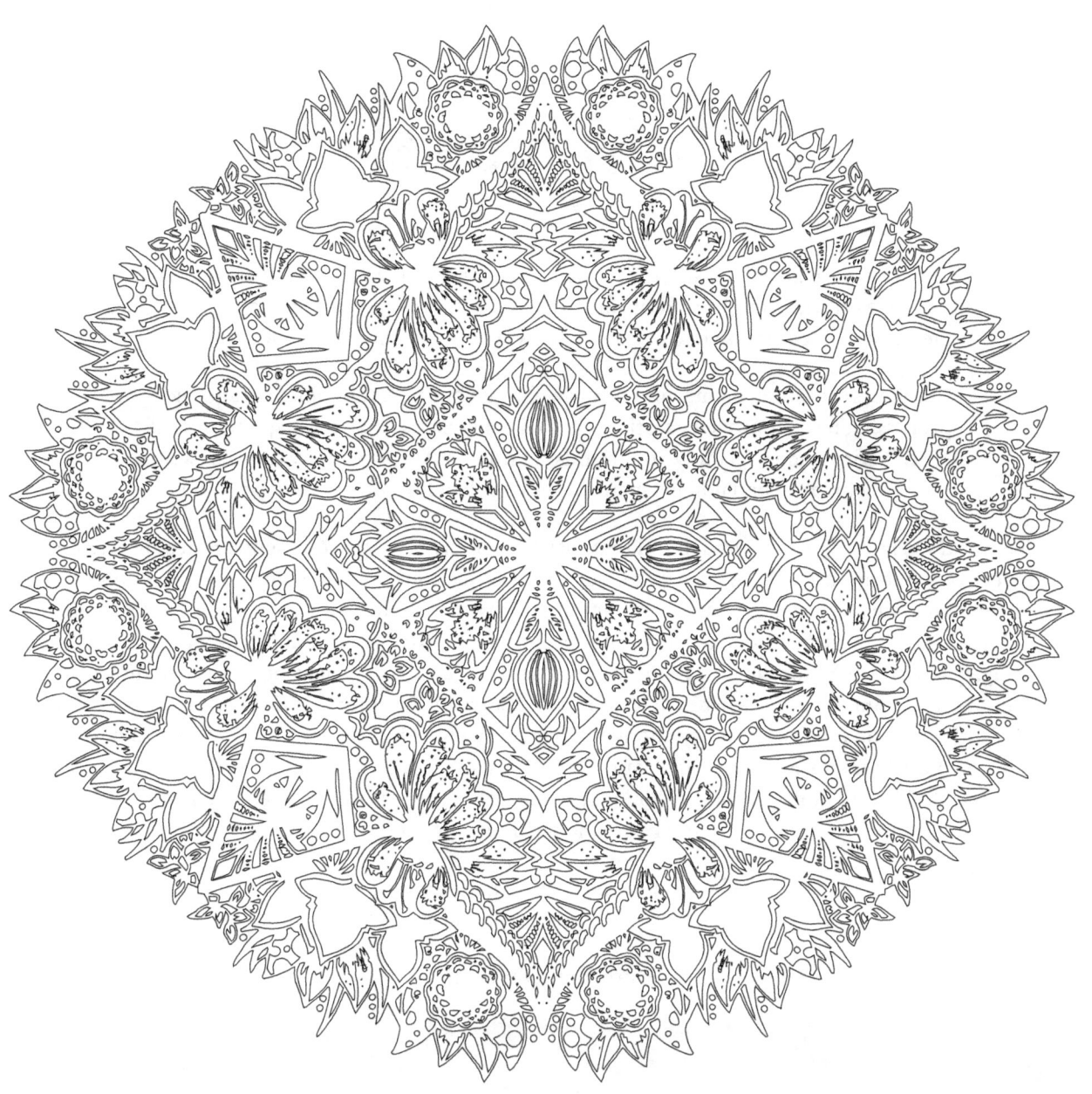

What now?

I hope these poems have given you some joy and comfort. My aim is to provide a little motivation and inspiration to move on with your life. Publishing this book has been an achievement for me, a goal that sometimes seemed impossible but one I knew would help me focus and look forward.

I still suffer from some mental and physical fatigue but my brain function and thought processing have improved greatly. These days I rarely write poems spontaneously but still write some for family and friends. I know that my creativity through writing has helped me and it helps many other people who suffer with depression.

I have always enjoyed exercise and found that focusing on my physical and mental fitness has helped my recovery enormously. There are a vast amount of services out there to help you with your fitness, so find a service and a trainer you want to spend time with. I found it was important to work with a personal trainer who understood me and my fatigue. I have been training now with Melinda Bingley and her team for the past 18 months and without doubt they have helped me to find 'me' after my stroke and focus on what I CAN do rather than what I cannot do. This has been invaluable and although you may not be lucky enough to live on the Sunshine Coast, head over to Melinda's website where there are a number of resources to help you on your way. Her ethos is 'making fitness fun' and I could not agree more. You may even find my fitness story under 'client stories.'
mabpersonaltraining.com.au

If you'd like to stay in touch and follow
my adventures, join me at:

astrokeofpoetry.com

A huge part of my recovery has depended on support from the National Stroke Foundation. They provided me with on line resources and literature with health and motivational advice to assist my recovery and specifically to aid me through my post stroke depression. They provide excellent verbal advice at StrokeLine Tel: 1800 787 653

The Foundation publish the twice-yearly newsletter
Stroke Connections which is a wonderful source of information and inspiration.
www.strokeconnection.strokeassociation.org

A recent addition to their resources is a free website filled with resources for stroke survivors, carers and family members. This site was developed in partnership with BUPA Health Foundation and a dedicated group of survivors, including myself as a pilot user. Carers have guided the Foundation to make this a one stop site for everything you need to know about stroke.
www.enableme.org.au

*Every book sold
raises funds for the
Stroke Foundation*

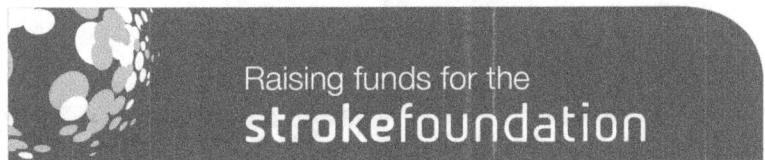

www.astrokeofpoetry.com

enableme is a world-first online platform

Goal setting is a great way to take charge of your own recovery.

FACE — Check their face. Has their mouth drooped?

ARMS — Can they lift both arms?

SPEECH — Is their speech slurred? Do they understand you?

TIME — Is critical. If you see any of these signs call 000 straight away.

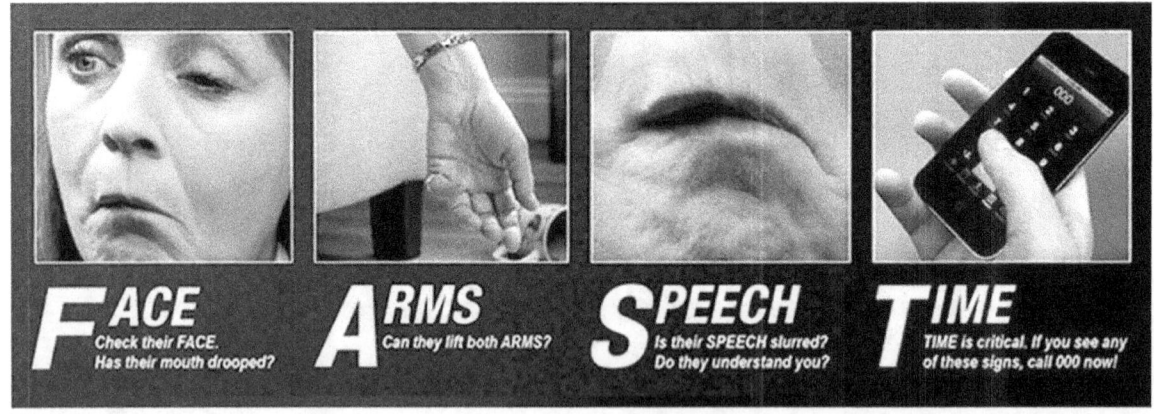

www.ingramcontent.com/pod-product-compliance
Lightning Source LLC
Chambersburg PA
CBHW080412300426
44113CB00015B/2497